THE VEIL OF ALLEGORY

MICHAEL MURRIN

The Veil of Allegory

SOME NOTES TOWARD A THEORY

OF ALLEGORICAL RHETORIC IN

THE ENGLISH RENAISSANCE

The University of Chicago Press

CHICAGO AND LONDON

Standard Book Number: 226-55400-7
Library of Congress Catalog Card Number: 69-19827
The University of Chicago Press, Chicago 60637
The University of Chicago Press, Ltd., London W.C. 1

To Jerome McGann

ἐμνήσθην δ' ὀσσάκις ἀμφότεροι
ἥλιον ἐν λέσχῃ κατεδύσαμεν

Contents

Introduction

NUMEROUS books have been published on Spenser recently and more are coming out. Most of these are close studies of his text. The purpose of this book is quite different. I have tried to step away from the poems and understand them generally as rhetoric. Everyone knows that poetry invariably had a rhetorical dimension in the Renaissance, but this fact has led to certain abuses in modern criticism. The rhetorical handbooks will not explain the structure and purpose of an allegory by themselves; they were designed for an essentially different rhetorical situation. To understand veiled communication a critic must explore a considerable variety of texts, which, though interdependent, are narrow and specific in their ends. He must draw out of this material a comprehensive theory of allegorical rhetoric. The result should be a book somewhat like Rosemond Tuve's studies in imagery: a general background will have been provided which will illuminate individual poems in an unforeseen way. I hope by this study to alter the kinds of questions which we ask of a text. I wish to stimulate controversy, to provoke thought. For this reason I have refrained from expressing my own interpretations as much as possible, using standard critics instead. A study designed to raise new issues should not kill them with detailed answers.

Although the argument of this book is rather complex, I have tried to write as clearly as I can. I have also tried to be brief. Citations are kept at a minimum, and there is little explicit controversy with contemporary critics. The argument of the book by itself is controversial enough. In an age where more is published than necessary, a scholar has a practical obligation to write less and say more. The style and method of this book represent an attempt in this direction.

This study, of course, serves various minor aims. To list some of them: I have tried to free Spenser from biblical exegesis and sketch out his late classical tradition of allegory; I have tried to suggest some of the ways in which Spenser relates to Donne; and I have tried to change our perspective on the major early critics in English: Sidney, Puttenham, and Jonson.

I wish to thank Howard K. Willett, whose foundation gave me much needed time and money to write this study. William Farrell and Jerome McGann read the manuscript as I wrote it, and I am dependent on them for many helpful suggestions. Their ideas have had considerable influence on my argument. I am indebted to David Bevington, who read the final draft, to William Ringler, who read parts of the manuscript, and to Charles Prouty. It was under his doctoral direction that I first began struggling with the problems of Spenser's language. I must also thank Mark Rosin, with whom I discussed most of my ideas.

A small portion of chapter 7 was read at a meeting of the Renaissance Seminar of the University of Chicago in the fall of 1966.

A last word. Since the method of this book precludes much explicit reference to the work of contemporary scholars, I would like to use this occasion to thank some of them: William Nelson and Thomas Roche for Spenser; Louis Martz and George Williamson for Donne; Rosemond Tuve, Frances Yates, Father Ong, and Marshall McLuhan for general background; Henri DeLubac for biblical exegesis; Eric Havelock, C. H. Dodd, and Gerhard von Rad for the antique sources. And that only begins the list.

Paul Alpers' *The Poetry of "The Faerie Queene"* came out, unfortunately, too late for me to use it. Although he is unconcerned with the question of oral poetry, his brilliant analysis of Spenser's formulaic style bears out my own contentions in that regard.

THE VEIL OF ALLEGORY

❧ 1 ❧

Allegory and Oratory

IN TUDOR ENGLAND poetry was commonly regarded as an oral art, but not in the modern sense of that term, for the poet did not create songs without a text by the formulaic technique Perry and Lord have found in Homer or the Yugoslav bards. He depended on a written text from which he read, but in theory his poem existed only when he actually spoke it. Ficino classifies poetry with music because the ear rather than the eye senses it, and Stephen Hawes in his discussion of poetry actually devotes some fifty lines to pronunciation.[1] The poet must speak with a humble and moderate voice; he must keep his accent and gestures refined and express in his face the joy or sadness of his tale. As a result of this theory the critics of poetry quite naturally looked to the rhetoricians for aid in their task, since the rhetoricians were professionally concerned with the problems of oral communication and poetry, after all, was a kind of rhetoric. The rhetorical manuals supplied the critic with a necessary precision of language; and it is in this area that contemporary scholars have accomplished much fruitful work since the last war. Unfortunately, the relationship of poetry to rhetoric has also caused considerable confusion, both in the sixteenth century and in the twentieth, mainly because of the Renaissance identification of poetry with allegory. The old handbooks of rhetoric were intended to describe oratory

NOTE: All quotations are taken from the standard critical editions, unless otherwise noted, and will not be cited in the footnotes.

[1] For Hawes, see *The Pastime of Pleasure*, ed. W. E. Mead, EETS (London, 1928), 1184–1239. For Ficino, see the *De divino furore* in the *Opera omnia*, reproduced by M. Sancipriano and presented by P. O. Kristeller (Turin, 1959), 1. 2. 612ff.

3

rather than allegory, and the two forms differ radically from each other as modes of communication. The problem becomes much worse for the modern critic, because formal English criticism practically begins with Sidney, Puttenham, and Jonson, three influential writers from the end of the period who rejected the traditional identification of poetry with allegory and tried to bring the poet closer to the orator. Thus, the modern critic will not find a real understanding of a poem like *The Faerie Queene* among the great critics of his own language and will be misled if he turns to rhetoricians like Wilson, Sherry, or Peacham. He will be further confused by the norms operative in the critical controversies which occurred at the end of Elizabeth's reign. Sidney, Puttenham, and later Jonson all rejected the kind of obscure style Spenser created for the allegory in his *Shepheardes Calender*, since they wanted the poet to write in a clear style—an idea appropriate for oratory but quite foreign to allegory. Therefore, the modern critic who wishes to understand the complex rhetorical function of an allegory like *The Faerie Queene* must first disentangle oratory and allegory before he can begin to find analogues and operative criteria for the "oral" poetry of Edmund Spenser.

In oratory the rhetor or speaker derives his arguments from the commonplace notions of his immediate audience. This principle applies to both ends of the spectrum formed by oratorical theory: that of logos, or rational persuasion, and that of pathos, or emotional persuasion. Aristotle and Cicero, who may be taken to represent these opposed conceptions of oratory, agree that the audience determines the kind of rhetoric adopted by the speaker on any occasion. For Aristotle, enthymemes or rhetorical syllogisms may constitute "the very body and substance of persuasion" (*Rhetoric* 1. 1),[2] but the rhetor derives his enthymemes from popular beliefs in his audience:

---

[2] All quotations from the *Rhetoric* are taken from Lane Cooper's translation (New York, 1960), with the omission of his bracketed additions to the text.

Even if our speaker has the most accurate scientific information, still there are persons whom he could not readily persuade with scientific arguments. True instruction, by the method of logic, is here impossible; the speaker must frame his proofs and arguments with the help of common knowledge and accepted opinions.

[*Rhetoric* 1. 1]

The orator may eventually lead his audience to new conclusions or identify their ideas with a particular issue or person, but in either case he must begin with popular ideas. Cicero, though arguing for pathos, has Antonius make the same point:[3]

Now nothing in oratory, Catulus, is more important than to win for the orator the favour of his hearer, and to have the latter so affected as to be swayed by something resembling a mental impulse or emotion, rather than by judgment or deliberation.

[*De oratore* 2. 42. 178]

The various styles of oratory, such as the Asiatic, Rhodian, or Attic, are determined by the taste of the audience. The "rich and unctuous diction" (*Orator* 7. 25) of the Asiatics pleases the unrefined ears of Asiatic Greeks but not those of Athens. As Cicero remarks in his own person:

The eloquence of orators has always been controlled by the good sense of the audience, since all who desire to win approval have regard to the goodwill of their auditors, and shape and adapt themselves completely according to this and to their opinion and approval.

[*Orator* 7. 24]

Aristotle sums up this principle laconically at the beginning of the second book of the *Rhetoric* when he says:

Now Rhetoric finds its end in judgment—for the audience judges the counsels that are given, and the decision is a judgment.

[3] All quotations from Cicero are taken from the Loeb translations.

The assumption holds true even for epideictic rhetoric, that middle ground between oratory and poetry. In this kind of oratory the speaker praises or blames a person or an object, as in a funeral sermon. One might expect different norms here, for Aristotle remarks that: "The style of epideictic speeches is the most literary, since it is meant to be read" (3. 12) and he considers the audience to be observers or critics of the speech itself instead of people who must make a decision on a particular issue (1. 3). When he discusses the virtues the orator must praise in a eulogy, however, he defines them according to popular opinion:

> Whatever the quality an audience esteems, the speaker must attribute that quality to the object of his praise, whether the audience be Scythians, or Spartans, or scholars. The rule is, whatever is esteemed is to be treated as noble, since the two things are nearly one in the popular view.
>
> [1. 9]

In another passage he is still more explicit: "And the same thing holds good of epideictic speaking; you compose your speech for an audience, and the audience is the 'judge'" (2. 18). Cicero ignores epideictic oratory, but Thomas Wilson in his *Arte of Rhetorike*, though he enumerates no principles, presupposes Aristotle's attitude. In one of his examples he argues that an orator can praise a person for his nationality, in which case English nationality surpasses the Scotch, and French the Irish—ideas certainly acceptable to a London audience but not to one in Edinburgh.[4] The audience exercises control over all forms of oratory, whether the deliberative and forensic, its practical forms, or its more literary mode, the epideictic.

From this basic assumption of audience control Cicero infers a second principle. If the audience controls the orator, it also controls the critic. The learned critic can only judge oratory by its effects: if an orator succeeds with his audience, he is good; if he fails, no profundity of thought or grace of diction can make

---

4 Thomas Wilson, *The Arte of Rhetorike* (London, 1567), f7ʳ.

him a good orator. The critic need not even hear what the orator says, he merely needs to observe his audience. The judgment of the audience and that of the critic must coincide:

> . . . this is the very mark of supreme oratory, that the supreme orator is recognized by the people. Thus, while Antigenidas the flutist may very well have said to a pupil, whom the public had listened to coldly, "play for me and for the Muses"; I would say rather to our Brutus here, addressing as he does commonly a great audience, "play for me and for the people, my dear Brutus." They will recognize the effect, I shall understand the reason for it.
>
> [*Brutus* 49. 186–87]

Unfortunately, the allegorical poet sometimes found himself in the position of the flutist while asked to perform the functions of an orator.

In matters of style, audience control expresses itself in the two principles of decorum and clarity. Decorum, which assumes so much importance in the poetics of Puttenham and other Renaissance theorists, requires no discussion here, since other scholars, like Rosemund Tuve in her *Elizabethan and Metaphysical Imagery* (1947), have already examined it in detail. The decorous speaker recognizes that the social status of his audience as well as his own position in the society will affect the language he uses. He must find the right words both for his subject matter and for the social occasion. Clarity, however, needs some explanation because it strikes at the heart of the confusion between oratory and poetry and was used as a club against Spenser. Aristotle again reduces this principle to a few words:

> We may therefore . . . regard it as settled that a good style is, first of all, clear. The proof is that language which does not convey a clear meaning fails to perform the very function of language.
>
> [*Rhetoric* 3. 2]

Thomas Wilson expresses the same idea: the orator can never

delight and consequently sway his audience unless he talks clearly.[5] Cicero regards the matter as so obvious that he has Crassus pass it over with a simple comment in the *De oratore* (3. 10. 38).

It is here that the gap between poetry and oratory becomes most apparent, because so much poetry is notoriously unclear— whether one thinks of the odes of Pindar, songs from the *Elder Edda*, or the poems of T. S. Eliot—and allegory is preeminently an obscure form of poetry. Critics like Jonson and Puttenham, who tend to identify the principles of poetry with those of oratory, would never allow for the allusive allegory and unnatural diction of *The Shepheardes Calender*. Puttenham paraphrases an elaborate passage from Wilson to reinforce his arguments for clarity in poetry. The poet must avoid any diction peculiar to a particular profession or to a group in a given area. Jonson gives it a historical perspective:[6]

> *Custome* is the most certaine Mistresse of Language, as the publicke stampe makes the current money. But wee must not be too frequent with the mint, every day coyning. Nor fetch words from the extreme and utmost ages; since the chiefe vertue of a style is perspicuitie, and nothing so vitious in it, as to need an Interpreter.

By this criterion Homer as well as Spenser must be denounced, for in both the poetic style does not reflect current idiom. They can be called unclear.

This identification of oratory and poetry came easily to those like Aristotle, who modeled their poetic theory on that mixed art form, the drama, though even here their principles eventually break down. The dramatist like the orator must concern himself with an immediate audience, one which includes people of different backgrounds, education, and tastes. If the audience misses

[5] Ibid., f1ᵛ-2ʳ.

[6] George Puttenham, *The Arte of English Poesie* 3. 4, pp. 144–45 in the Willcock and Walker edition; Ben Jonson, *Discoveries*, p. 622 in Herford and Simpson's *Ben Jonson* (Oxford, 1947), vol. 8 (hereafter referred to as *Discoveries* HS8).

some lines, they cannot be repeated or explained later, and the dramatic effect of the whole play is accordingly diminished. Therefore, clarity becomes a practical necessity for the dramatist and applies as a norm to the stage as well as to the forum and the lawcourts. Aristotle uses the same *general* criteria of style indifferently for oratory and poetry,[7] and Jonson tried to be clear in his poetry as well as in his comedies. There is some drama, however, which violates the principle of clarity. Aeschylus and the later Shakespeare are not praised for their lucidity. The principle cannot explain all drama, because the dramatist, insofar as he is a poet, assumes different basic criteria. The audience affects but does not control his rhetoric, for his primary commitment is to the truth or matter he is attempting to express. This commitment controls the allegorical poet in a much more extreme fashion, since he expends much of his energy in protecting his truth from the multitude rather than in communicating it. In this sense a poet like Spenser obeys norms directly contrary to those of the orator and constructs what one might call a kind of antirhetoric. Cicero, by his anecdote about Antimachus, finely characterizes the crucial difference between the poet's and the orator's attitude toward his audience:

> Demosthenes could never have said what is reported of the famous poet Antimachus. When reading that long and well-known poem of his before an assembled audience, in the very midst of his reading all his listeners left him but Plato: "I shall go on reading," he said, "just the same; for me Plato alone is as good as a hundred thousand." And quite right; for a poem full of obscure allusions can from its nature only win the approbation of the few; an oration meant for a general public must aim to win the assent of the throng. If Demosthenes on the other hand had held only Plato as his auditor and was deserted by the rest, he could not have uttered a single word.
>
> [*Brutus* 51. 191]

7 *Rhetoric* 3. 2. In the preceding chapter, however, Aristotle on more specific grounds distinguishes the language of the poet from that of the orator.

One must never allow a similar interest in the problems of oral communication or a common technical language to blur this essential difference between the orator and the poet. The one plays for the expert and the crowd; the other, for the expert and the Muses.

Truth rather than popular belief provides the allegorical poet with his operative control as it also does the philosopher. Nashe defines poetry in these terms: "I account of Poetrie as of a more hidden and diuine kinde of Philosophy, enwrapped in blinde Fables and darke stories." In his *Genealogie deorum gentilium* Boccaccio distinguishes this allegorical poetry from philosophy by its mode of expression. The philosopher discovers truth through syllogistic discourse; the poet protects truth by the veil of allegory.[8] In similar fashion he separates allegory from oratory: "Yet, in truth, among the disguises of fiction rhetoric has no part, for whatever is composed as under a veil, and thus exquisitely wrought, is poetry and poetry alone" (*GDG* 14. 7). Truth demands darkness: the veil of allegory indicates the presence of truth and simultaneously gives to the definition of poetry its specific difference.

By means of the veil the poet performs three related functions for his audience. Sometimes the poet thinks himself obliged to keep the multitude from debasing truth:

> . . . where matters truly solemn and memorable are too much exposed, it is his office by every effort to protect as well as he can and remove them from the gaze of the irreverent, that they cheapen not by too common familiarity.
>
> [*GDG* 14. 12]

Or in Harington's words: "that they might not be rashly abused by prophane wits, in whom science is corrupted, like good wine

---

[8] For Nashe, see G. Gregory Smith, *Elizabethan Critical Essays* (Oxford, 1964), 1: 328. For Boccaccio, see the *Genealogie deorum gentilium* 14. 17; in vol. 2 of Romano's edition (Bari, 1951). My quotations from the *Genealogie* are taken from Osgood's translation in his *Boccaccio on Poetry* (Indianapolis, 1956).

in a bad vessell."⁹ Harington's statement also suggests the rationale behind the second function of the veil. In certain instances the veil exists in the minds of the audience, not in the language of the poet, for some truths are so profound that, though expressed in the clearest terms, they will appear obscure to most people:

> . . . when things perfectly clear seem obscure, it is the beholder's fault. To a half-blind man, even when the sun is shining its brightest, the sky looks cloudy. Some things are naturally so profound that not without difficulty can the most exceptional keenness in intellect sound their depths; like the sun's globe, by which, before they can clearly discern it, strong eyes are sometimes repelled.
>
> [GDG 14. 12]

In his prologues and dedicatory sonnets to *The Faerie Queene*, Spenser combines these two functions of the veil. To Burleigh he says that he deliberately veiled his "deeper sence" from the "comune vew," using Boccaccio's first explanation. But in the Prologue to Book Two he turns the position around. The reality of the Queen, like the sun, blinds—so he enfolds her light in a veil "That feeble eyes your glory may behold" (Pro. 5). He substitutes for the veil in the minds of his audience his own veil, through which the sun may at least shine, though faintly. This is the third function of the veil in Boccaccio, one which grows out of the second. The poet covers the sun with clouds, through which people may see its light, though they cannot tell its exact position. The few, however, can with difficulty pierce the cloud bank and see the truth, and this is the most important function of the veil. It makes truth valuable for a few people in the poet's audience. In oral communication truth has no power; the speaker must make it valuable for his auditors. The veil of allegory creates the value truth needs by setting up difficulties for the understanding:

⁹ In Smith, 2: 203.

Surely no one can believe that poets invidiously veil the truth with fiction, either to deprive the reader of the hidden sense, or to appear the more clever; but rather to make truths which would otherwise cheapen by exposure the object of strong intellectual effort and various interpretation, that in ultimate discovery they shall be more precious.

[GDG 14. 12]

The teacher who spends an hour making his class discover an old cliché which he could have explained in five minutes uses a similar principle. The auditor must buy his pearl at great price.

For this very reason Renaissance critics sometimes attacked the philosophers. They denuded truth, consequently truth lost its value, and a society where truth is not honored can only decline. As Harington says: "Indeed it hath bene thought by men of verie good iudgement, such manner of Poeticall writing was an excellent way to preserue all kinde of learning from that corruption which now it is come to since they left that mysticall writing of verse."[10] Henry Reynolds in the beginning of his *Mythomystes* (1632) speaks apocalyptically:[11]

I haue thought vpon the times wee liue in, and am forced to affirme the world is decrepit, and, out of its age & doating estate, subiect to all the imperfections that are inseparable from that wracke and maime of Nature, that the young behold with horror, and the sufferers thereof lye vnder with murmur and languishment. Euen the generall Soule of this great Creature, whereof euery one of ours is a seuerall peece, seemes bedrid, as vpon her deathbed and neere the time of her dissolution to a second better estate and being; the yeares of her strength are past, and she is now nothing but disease, for the Soules health is no other then meerely the knowledge of the Truth of things: Which health the worlds youth inioyed, and hath now exchanged for it all the diseases of all errors, heresies, and different sects and schismes of opinions and vnderstandings in all matter of Arts, Sciences,

10 Ibid.

11 In J. E. Spingarn, *Critical Essays of the Seventeenth Century* (Bloomington, 1957), 1: 144-45.

and Learnings whatsoeuer. To helpe on these diseases to incurability, what age hath euer beene so fruitfull of libertv in all kindes, and of all permission and allowance for this reason of ours, to runne wildely all her owne hurtfullest wayes without bridle, bound, or limit at all? For instance, what bookes haue wee of what euer knowledge, or in what mysteries soeuer, wisely by our Auncients (for auoiding of this present malady the world is now falne into) couched and carefully infoulded, but must bee by euery illiterate person without exception deflowred and broke open, or broke in pieces, because beyond his skill to vnlocke them?

Reynolds has been reading Giovanni Pico della Mirandola and has learned the language of the Hellenistic mystagogue. Allegory, by veiling truth, preserves the health of human society, and the rending of the veil relates somehow to the decay of the cosmos. This mystical conception of truth and value escapes the normal techniques of investigation available to the rhetorician. The Florentine Platonists had literally revived all the ancient theories of allegory and mystery common in the Roman Empire, and their ideas captured the imaginations of many in England. Later we must go into their theories more deeply; now, our concern is with the effects of veiled truth on the poet's audience.

The allegorical poet affects his audience more in the manner of a Hebrew prophet than in that of a classical orator. Instead of appealing to all the people and attempting to win them over to a particular point of view, the poet causes a division in his audience, separating the few from the many, those who understand from those who cannot, much like Cicero's Antimachus, who ended up addressing Plato alone in an empty hall. The auditor's capacity for profound thought determines his position, and sometimes the critics accordingly multiply the divisions in the audience to make them correspond to the levels of meaning they have found in allegory. Harington has three divisions and three levels: literal, moral, and allegorical:[12]

[12] In Smith, 2: 203.

For the weaker capacities will feede themselues with the pleasantnes of the historie and sweetnes of the verse, some that haue stronger stomackes will as it were take a further taste of the Morall sence, a third sort, more high conceited then they, will digest the Allegorie.

Whatever the number of divisions, the allegory proper remains the property of the inner group, whether there are one or more outside circles.

Harington's distinction likewise helps one to distinguish allegory from morality drama and from the popular literature of ethical instruction. A play like *Mankind*, for example, performs the function of a popular sermon and is obviously designed for a wide audience. It contains no deep truths, but simply stresses certain aspects of Christian morality. In Harington's terms it would not be an allegory at all, since it expresses no philosophical perspective. The same applies to Puritan polemics and to similar literature written for the ordinary citizen. Although a modern might class them as allegories, Harington, Spenser, and those in the late classical tradition of allegory would not call them so. As Henry Reynolds remarks in *Mythomystes*, moral instruction requires no concealment.[13] Such art obeys the laws of oratory and never depends upon an elite audience. There is no inner circle.

The norms for the elite audience to whom the poet primarily speaks are both aristocratic and academic. Spenser designs his *Faerie Queene* for an upper class audience: "The generall end therefore of all the booke is to fashion a gentleman or noble person in vertuous and gentle discipline," and he sings "of Knights and Ladies gentle deeds"; but he also calls his audience the Muse's "learned throng," combining aristocratic and academic criteria. Natalis Comes does not think that fables help any but those with natural genius.[14] The critics put the greatest

13 In Spingarn, 1: 155, 162.
14 The Letter to Raleigh and *FQ* 1. Pro. 1. The portrait of a gentleman might be of use to a lawyer imitating the mores of the upper classes, but it would not help a peasant—or most lawyers, for that matter. For Natalis Comes, see the *Mythologiae* (Venice, 1568) 1. 2. f4ᵛ.

stress on academic qualifications; Boccaccio's reader is a modern graduate student:

> But I repeat my advice to those who would appreciate poetry, and unwind its difficult involutions. You must read, you must persevere, you must sit up nights, you must inquire, and exert the utmost power of your mind. If one way does not lead to the desired meaning, take another; if obstacles arise, then still another; until, if your strength holds out, you will find that clear which at first looked dark. For we are forbidden by divine command to give that which is holy to dogs, or to cast pearls before swine.
>
> [GDG 14. 12]

A man had to recognize in allegory a specialized form of discourse, something which demanded of him an unusual mode of thought. Otherwise, despite whatever natural qualifications he might have, he would react to a poem in an ignorant manner. Lodge complains that Gosson is a *"homo literatus*, a man of the letter, little sauoring of learning."[15] Men like Gosson, educated in their own fields, represented a real danger to poetry, for they tried to read and judge it without the proper credentials. Boccaccio most viciously attacks the lawyers, sensing the aggression of one profession toward another. Spenser advises those who judge *The Faerie Queene* "th' aboundance of an idle braine":

> Of Faerie lond yet if he more inquire,
> By certaine signes here set in sundry place
> He may it find; ne let him then admire,
> But yield his sence to be too blunt and bace,
> That no'te without an hound fine footing trace.
>
> [FQ 2. Pro. 1, 4]

The poet did not completely ignore the majority of his audience. Although he excluded them from truth by the veil of allegory, he yet wished to entertain them. In Horatian terms, he gave profit to the few and pleasure to the many. Only extreme obscurantists like Antimachus chased the many out of the lecture hall; most poets preferred to effect a silent, painless division

15 In Smith, 1: 65.

in their audience. The Horatian norms, of course, do not exactly
fit the situation of the allegorical poet, for Horace was talking
in terms of the drama, in which the poet had to attract both
young and old. The equation *the old = the few, the young =
the many* did work, however, after a rough fashion. Horace describes the typical young man in a way which would accurately
characterize the allegorist's conception of the many:[16]

> The beardless youth, finally free of his guardian,
> Rejoices in horses and hounds and the sun-drenched grass
> Of the Campus Martius: he is putty in your hands to mold
> To evil courses, resentful of warning advisers. . . .
>   [*Ars poetica* 161-63]

He lacks wisdom, and, Platonically, lives solely in a sense world,
like the multitude.

These Horatian ideas make possible for the poet a more positive attitude toward the many. The separation of his audience
need not be absolute; some young men from among the many,
charmed by the allegorical story, might be encouraged to study
and understand it: "[poetry] pleaseth fooles, and so pleaseth
them that, if they marke it and obserue it well, it will in time
make them wise."[17] In such a situation the poet by his rhetoric
draws out of the many those youths with sufficient natural gifts
and brings them over to the elite; the poet becomes an ideal
educator, particularly in regard to biblical studies, the revelation
at the basis of Renaissance society. Boccaccio always assumed
that the Christian revelation took an essentially literary form,
identifying scriptural *figurae* with poetic allegory. Consequently,
there could be no better introduction to scriptural theology than
poetry, as Harington says:[18]

> [Biblical mysteries are] not subiect to euerie weake capacitie,
> no nor to the highest wits and iudgments, except they be

---

[16] The translation is Bovie's in his *Satires and Epistles of Horace*
(Chicago, 1963).
[17] Harington, in Smith, 2: 207.
[18] In Smith, 2: 198.

first illuminat by Gods spirit or instructed by his teachers and preachers: therefore we do first read some other authors, making them as it were a looking glasse to the eyes of our minde, and then after we haue gathered more strength, we enter into profounder studies of higher mysteries, hauing first as it were enabled our eyes by long beholding the sunne in a bason of water at last to looke vpon the sunne it selfe.

The scriptural analogy introduces a new element into this discussion of audience criteria, for it adds a moral dimension to the poet's activity.

Platonists converted the few and the many into the good and the bad. John Rainolds quotes the *Alcibiades*, saying that poets wrapped golden thoughts in the obscuring folds of enigma so only the good might understand.[19] Henry Reynolds in *Mythomystes* uses "Orpheus" for the same purpose:

> O you that vertue follow, to my sense
> Bend your attentiue minds; Prophane ones, hence!

Earlier he repeats Pico's arguments that few can perceive Intellectual Beauty, because few can escape the body. Ficino explains the philosophic basis for this separation:[20]

> As a dirty vessel makes dirty by its contagion whatsoever fluid, even the sweetest, you may pour into it, so a bad mind when receiving knowledge produces malice, not wisdom. Moreover, as the air is related to the light of the sun, so is the mind to the light of truth and wisdom. Consequently, neither the air nor the intellect ever receives its rays while clouded, and each receives them directly so soon as it becomes pure and serene. . . . Purify the eyes of reason from all dirt of this unwholesome body; turn away the glance of the mind from the shadow of the lowest matter; direct the sight of inner intelligence toward the light of the higher

[19] John Rainolds, *Oratio in laudem artis poeticae*, ed. W. Ringler, translated by Walter Allen (Princeton, 1940), p. 41.

[20] For Reynolds see Spingarn, 1: 168, 151. Ficino is quoted by P. O. Kristeller in the *Philosophy of Marsilio Ficino*, translated by Virginia Conant (New York, 1943), pp. 301-2. I have omitted his bracketed insertions. For Harington, see Smith, 2: 203.

form. By that same source from which matter when sufficiently prepared is first suddenly shaped into corporeal forms, the mind when sufficiently disposed is at once endowed with incorporeal forms. And as it is illumined by the clear rays of truth, so its cup runs over with true joy.

Harington similarly talks of "good wine in a bad vessell." The Platonist equates knowledge with virtue, the academic with the moral, and extends the *differentiae* to the allegorical form itself. The multitude can imagine the scenes described by the poets; they can visualize Phaëton losing control of the Sun's horses, but they cannot understand the sense of the story. They remain prisoners of the "Body," of the sensible world, and have no Mind. Consequently, they have no virtue.

Morally the poet takes upon himself a role like that of the prophet: "Indeed Prophets and Poets haue been thought to haue a great affinitie, as the name *Vates* in Latin doth testifie."[21] By his allegorical discourse the poet makes the good and creates evil in his audience, separating the sheep from the goats. As with the prophet, the people judge themselves by their reactions to his discourse. Both the prophet and the poet find their operative control in truth, and both fail in their mission by the standards of oratory. The failure of Jeremiah to make the people hear his truth anticipates the failure of Antimachus, who could keep only one auditor. Both the allegorist and the prophet address the many but succeed only with the few.

The hierophant of the ancient mysteries provides a still closer analogy to the role of the allegorical poet, one recognized both by modern critics and by Renaissance theorists, who borrowed his language. Unlike his twentieth-century successors, the critic of the fifteenth or sixteenth century did not have the sciences of archeology and anthropology to help him understand the worship of Isis, Demeter, and Mithra; he had to depend upon the writers of the Roman Empire from the early days of Philo, Clement, and Apuleius to the last period of the pagan revival,

[21] Harington, in Smith, 2: 205.

when the Emperor Julian and Sallustius tried to formalize the criticism of ritual myth. All these writers saw in the mystery religions an excellent justification for the techniques of exclusive allegory. The analogy becomes particularly close in the case of the Orphic religion, which drew its ritual from the allegorical poetry of its founder. The hierophant of the mysteries habitually classified people into the categories of the sacred and the profane, the initiate and the uninitiate, those who know the secrets of salvation and those who do not. In defense of truth he excluded outsiders from his dramatic rituals and did not allow the initiate to reveal his secrets to the "profanum vulgus," much as the Renaissance poet veiled truth from the eyes of the many. Through dramatic ritual the hierophant converted truth into value, for he cloaked truth in ceremony and darkness and gave to it a power it could not have outside its ritual context. His worshipers went through a profound but controlled psychological experience of truth, which approximated the act of dying, the final and ultimate ordeal of all men. The votary of the god first wandered about in darkness, wearily hurrying back and forth, and then encountered the terror of initiation with amazement, trembling, and sweating. In this dark hour he perceived a sudden blaze of light and entered into the grassy fields of Elysium, where he joined the crowned figures of the initiated and heard the music and song of Paradise.[22] This experience of death lent truth an absolute psychological value, something which the worshiper could never share with the outsider, who still feared to die. The hierophant placed truth beyond the range of normal human life and therefore made it priceless.

It is in the two figures of the prophet and the priest that one learns the antique background of allegorical rhetoric and gains some insight into its operation. For the priest we will use Pico della Mirandola as our guide, for we need a specifically Renaissance understanding of the mysteries. It was the circle of the

[22] Paraphrased from Themistios, quoted by George Mylonas in *Eleusis and the Eleusinian Mysteries* (Princeton, 1961), pp. 264-65.

Florentine Platonists which revived all these conceptions, influenced many writers of the sixteenth century, and in particular developed for allegory a philosophical and psychological justification beyond the reach of the ordinary critic. They could never have successfully revived the viewpoint of the mysteries, however, if it had not already been implicit in the rhetoric of Renaissance allegory.

2

Allegory and Prophecy in the Ancient World

And I saw heaven opened, and behold a white
horse; and he that sat upon him was called Faithful
and True. . . . And he was clothed with a vesture
dipped in blood: and his name is called The Word
of God.

[Rev. 19:11–13]

And Dionysiac truth appropriates the entire realm
of myth as symbolic language for its own insights,
which it expresses partly in the public rite of tragedy and partly in the secret celebrations of dramatic
mysteries, but always under the old mythic veil.

[*Birth of Tragedy* 10]

BEFORE BEGINNING a discussion of such a wide subject as ancient
allegory and prophecy, it is necessary to delimit the argument.
The purpose of this analysis is roughly twofold. First of all, a
modern needs to recover the conception of antiquity held by
many writers and theorists of the Renaissance. Such a viewpoint
is distinctly not modern, nor was it held by everyone in the Renaissance. Then as now one could draw diametrically opposed conclusions from the same texts. Were Homer's epics popular or
elitist? Were Christ's parables designed for popular instruction
or used to exclude the ordinary man from any real understanding? Such questions are debatable, but the concern here is solely
with one side of the problem—the elitist interpretations. The
second purpose of this chapter is historical. Pico della Mirandola

and others did not fabricate their understanding of antiquity out of nothing. Their interpretations were carefully derived from the texts themselves and from ancient criticism of those texts. Their theories are not just historical facts for a student of culture but are worthy of consideration for their own sake, even in the twentieth century.

I

In the ancient world the prophet and the allegorist both practiced a kind of exclusive rhetoric. They created in their audience divisions and sharply different reactions, because they were committed first and last to the truth they had received through divine inspiration and could not appeal to popular opinion. The two differed in the manner in which they brought about this separation in their audience. The allegorist decided ahead of time the principles which would divide the few from the many; he presupposed such a division, which automatically occurred whenever he spoke. He tried to exclude the many from the understanding of truth, though not from its proclamation. He discovered the appropriate vehicle for truth in myth, parable, and apocalyptic vision, which the many could follow as a story but could never interpret properly. The vision never meant what it said; the proclamation itself became enigmatic, metaphorically comparable to the sphinxes guarding Egyptian temples, familiar symbols of the difficult and obscure. The prophet, without any prior assumptions, created rather than predetermined a separation in his audience. He came to divide father from son, mother from daughter; he was a stumbling block and a sign of contradiction to his own people. He spoke in a simple fashion, but his words burned, refining the good and consuming the bad. He talked to all men, but few listened to him: "Who hath believed our report?"[1] The prophet often found himself isolated, conversing

[1] Isa. 53:1. All biblical quotations are taken from the Authorized Version.

with a few faithful followers, like Jesus with the Apostles at the Last Supper, or completely alone, like Jeremiah in Egypt. He failed to convince the people of his truth, and his very failure justified the assumption of the allegorist: the many cannot receive truth. The prophet of one generation gives way to the visionary of the next; the clear flame disappears in smoke. Or the same transition could occur within a lifetime: Christ, as Matthew presents him, first tried prophetic rhetoric and after its failure resorted to the parabolic discourse of the allegorist.

The story of Jeremiah's Temple Sermon represents clearly all the relevant particulars of the prophet's rhetorical dilemma (Jeremiah 26). The word of the Lord came to Jeremiah at the beginning of Jehoiakim's reign (609-608 B.C.). He was ordered to stand in the court of the Temple and speak to all the Israelites who came to worship there; his purpose was a general reformation of the people, necessary to avert a catastrophe threatening the land, an invasion by the Babylonian armies which actually took place some years later. In a time of political and military crisis, one would normally expect from a speaker an extensive analysis of the current situation and an attempt to persuade the people to adopt a specific course of action. Jeremiah should have argued, if he were a classical rhetorician, that the Egyptian occupation of Syria could not last, that they could never defeat the Babylonian army in the field, and that the moral reformation of the people, begun by Josiah, had not been carried on by Jehoiakim. But Jeremiah did none of these things, for he had to be faithful to the word of the Lord which he had received, and that word was couched in extremely simplistic terms. Jeremiah only said that the people must listen to the Lord, obey the Law, and follow the commands of his prophets, which they had not done previously. The alternative was absolute ruin; the Lord promised to destroy the Temple as he had destroyed his old tabernacle at Shiloh long ago in the days of the Judges. This speech produced anything but agreement; the people, especially the priests and the other prophets, wanted to put Jeremiah to death, the punishment required for false prophecy. He had violated one of their basic assumptions when he threatened the Temple with destruction; for, since Jerusalem had survived the invasion of Sennacherib a century before, the Jews had believed that the Lord would never allow his city and Temple to be destroyed. Jeremiah had contradicted one of the most important commonplaces in the Jewish tradition.

At the trial which followed, Jeremiah answered the charge of false prophecy by a claim of divine inspiration. The people must listen to the Lord speaking through him or ruin would follow. He added a threat: if the Jews executed him, they would be liable for innocent blood and would have directly affronted their God. His argument convinced the princes and saved his life. In itself it functions merely as a counterclaim. The priests had charged that he prophesied falsely; he said he prophesied truly. This argument worked partially because the content of his message actually corresponded to the content of earlier prophetic utterances. The elders explained to the people that the prophet Micah had said much the same thing under King Hezekiah a century earlier, and the King and the people had listened to him. More typical, however, was the career of Jeremiah's contemporary Urijah, who spoke in the same terms and could not escape the death penalty. Having angered Jehoiakim, he fled into Egypt; but Jehoiakim sent envoys there and had him extradited. On his return he was slain with a sword and his body cast into the graves reserved for the common people. Jeremiah escaped this fate by his own defense and through the influence of a powerful friend, Ahikam the son of Shaphan.

The most astonishing aspect of this story is Jeremiah's own rhetoric. In a tense political crisis Jeremiah is trying to reach all the people by his speech, but he avoids all the standard devices of propaganda and oratory and reduces his message to a simple, either-or statement: repent or perish. Even the expanded text of his sermon which one finds in chapter 7 does not show anything more than an ornamental expansion of this simple proclamation.

The prophet does not trouble the people with refined distinctions or a variety of alternatives; instead he makes a final decision automatic, for the people cannot respond partially to such a demand. No middle position is allowed; the people must choose absolutely for one or the other side. In this case they choose to reject the prophet and practically kill him. Judgment has been passed automatically by the people on themselves, for, by their rejection of Yahweh's word, they reject his mercy. The prophet comes bringing light to the world and wants to lead his people out of the darkness. He comes with a positive mission; he wishes to save people, not to damn them. But his words have the opposite result. The people usually reject his words and become liable to judgment, for the words themselves have defined the consequences which follow from negative choice: in this case the Temple will be destroyed.[2] In the Renaissance, George Herbert applied this conception of the judging word to sermons; he has his parson warn the people: "that Sermons are dangerous things, that none goes out of Church as he came in, but either better, or worse; that none is careless before his Judg, and that the word of God shal judge us" (*Priest to the Temple* 7). Even the princes do not accept Jeremiah's message; they intervene in his favor because they think that a prophet should be allowed to speak Yahweh's word, not because they agree with Jeremiah.

On this occasion Jeremiah completely failed to persuade the people that they must change their ways, nor did he have more success in other sermons. Through his whole life the people never listened to him, not even after the stones of the Temple lay scattered in the city streets. Hence the emotional depression and gloomy atmosphere in his writings, as in many of the prophets. Jeremiah in one place complains that he is hated more than a usurer. Everyone curses him, and he wishes that he had never been born, for he is "a man of strife and a man of contention

---

[2] The explanation and metaphors are taken from John 12:46-48, where the same problem is explicitly discussed.

to the whole earth" (15:10). The people did not always reject
the prophet, as the elder remembers in the Temple Sermon.
Micah preached the same message a century before, and the
people listened to him. The writer of the Jonah story imagines
another total success; all Nineveh repented on Jonah's cry: "Yet
forty days, and Nineveh shall be overthrown" (3:4). The good
kings, David and Hezekiah, listened to their prophets. But the
career of Jeremiah's contemporary, Urijah ben Shemaiah, is
more typical. Jerusalem was a tomb for more prophets than
Christ. All of them provoked such hostility by their words that
they feared death. Their rhetoric alienated rather than convinced. The prophetic movement is a record of constant failure:

> Since the day that your fathers came forth out of the land
> of Egypt unto this day I have sent unto you all my servants
> the prophets, daily rising up early and sending them: yet
> they hearkened not unto me, nor inclined their ear, but hard-
> ened their neck: they did worse than their fathers.
> Therefore thou shalt speak all these words unto them; but
> they will not hearken to thee: thou shalt also call unto them;
> but they will not answer thee. But thou shalt say unto them,
> "This is a nation that obeyeth not the voice of the LORD
> their God, nor receiveth correction: truth is perished, and is
> cut off from their mouth."
>
> [Jer. 7:25-28]

The prophet at best might expect to cause a schism in his
audience; the princes at least did not oppose Jeremiah. In the
Bread of Life Discourse (John 7) Jesus at least does not lose
the Twelve, though even they include a traitor. The Athenians
mocked Paul: "Howbeit certain men clave unto him, and believed: among the which was Dionysius the Areopagite, and a
woman named Damaris, and others with them" (Acts 17:34).
The prophet finally rejects the people as they have rejected him
and turns to these faithful few: Christ gave to his Apostles "even
the Spirit of truth; whom the world cannot receive, because it
seeth him not, neither knoweth him" (John 14:17). The prophet
reserves his inspired truth for those willing to accept it. They

alone can receive the mercy and salvation offered by the prophet, as only the disciples saw the risen Christ. For the rest their wrath against the prophets provokes God's wrath against themselves; the separation becomes complete:

> Therefore have I hewed them by the prophets:
> I have slain them by the words of my mouth.
>> [Hos. 6:5]

In another episode Matthew has Christ pronounce the final rejection of the people in the very Temple courts. He curses the scribes and pharisees and finally Jerusalem itself, she who kills the prophets and stones them and will soon eliminate him (Matthew 23). The judgment consists of the destruction of the city, as it did in the days of Jeremiah, who advises the people to cut their hair in mourning and lament in the high places, "for the LORD hath rejected and forsaken the generation of his wrath" (7:29). Rejection by the people is judgment by God.

Writers define this conception of the word-as-separator with metaphors which they take from natural phenomena and from battle. The psalmist compares the word of God to a wind which brings winter and spring, life and death: the same agent has opposite effects. His word makes the snow fall thickly and scatters hoarfrost like ashes and brings terrible cold; but it also melts the ice, brings the spring breezes, and makes the waters flow again (Ps. 147:15-18). The prophets themselves frequently speak of the word as fire: "I will make my words in thy mouth fire, and this people wood, and it shall devour them" (Jer. 5:14). " 'Is not my word like as a fire,' saith the LORD; 'and like a hammer that breaketh the rock in pieces?' " (Jer. 23:29). But the fire could save as well as kill. For Luke, the Spirit comes in tongues of flame and the sound of a mighty wind and brings to all the disciples the knowledge of every language. By the same speech Peter addresses all the Jews of the Diaspora in their own dialects and tongues. In this Pentecost description Luke combines the images of wind and fire and equates them with Spirit, for the word is the medium of the spirit. Another such combination is the fire in the furnace which burned the Chaldeans outside but within was "as it had been a moist whistling wind" (Dan. 3:50 in the Apocrypha). The storm theophanies of Yahweh probably provided the original situation in which fire and wind could be identified: He rides the storm winds and lightens from the clouds, as does Baal.[3] The Johannine equivalent is the light shining in the darkness, announced in the Prologue and developed thematically throughout the whole gospel: "And the light shineth in darkness; and the darkness comprehended it not" (1:5). Light divides the darkness; therefore, it judges. Before, when all were in the darkness, no judgment or separation was possible, because all shared in the same condition. Once the light shines and salvation is offered, the people must choose between the darkness and the light, between salvation and judgment. Those who choose the light come there because they know that their deeds will bear the light of day, while those who remain in darkness want their actions concealed (John 3:20-21). People, therefore, indicate their moral condition by their choice: the good choose the light; the evil, the darkness. The prophet's word actually does create good and evil in his audience. Before he spoke, all shared in a sort of moral neutrality; afterward, they are morally divided.

Still another popular metaphor was that of the sword, which both defends and kills. In apocalyptic allegory the Spirit of Prophecy appears as the Word of God on a white horse: "And out of his mouth goeth a sharp sword, that with it he should smite the nations" (Rev. 19:15). The author of the Wisdom of Solomon explains the symbol: the Word of the Lord leaps down into the land of Egypt like a fierce man of war, bringing death to Israel's enemies by the sharp sword of his command

[3] For a fuller discussion of the prophetic word, see Gerhard von Rad, *Old Testament Theology*, translated by D. M. G. Stalker (New York, 1965), 2: 80-98; and C. H. Dodd, *The Interpretation of the Fourth Gospel* (Cambridge, 1963), pp. 263-85.

and, therefore, effects the salvation of the Jews. The release of
the Israelites from Egypt depends upon the Angel of Death, who
simultaneously glorifies the Jews and kills their oppressors
(18:7-16). Again, the same agent causes opposite effects. Another
analogy is water, which saves the thirsty and drowns the enemy,
the archetypes being the Deluge and the Passage of the Red
Sea.[4] In all these metaphors the same word can save or destroy,
as the prophet, whenever he speaks, brings the hour of judgment
to his people ('érchetai 'óra kaì nûn 'estín).[5] But, more important,
these metaphors indicate the cause of the prophet's own dilemma. The power of the word is God's, not the prophet's.
Yahweh himself makes his words fire, he himself brings winter
and spring, it is his word which divides the darkness and rides a
white horse: the prophet functions merely as his medium.

Prophecy cannot exist without inspiration. Deuteronomy
prescribes the death penalty for anyone who prophesies falsely,
that is, speaks by himself. Jeremiah, Isaiah, and Paul carefully
recount for their audiences the manner in which they received
the Word, for without it they have no authority.[6] Jeremiah is
particularly explicit. Yahweh wants to ordain him a prophet, but
Jeremiah, like Moses, objects that he has no speaking ability.
God replies that he will tell Jeremiah what to say and will give
him the courage necessary to face a hostile audience. He then
touches the mouth of the prophet and says: "Behold, I have put
my words in thy mouth" (1:9). Yahweh sets his prophet over
nations and kingdoms, to root them up and to pull them down,
to build and to plant. Now only Yahweh can pull down nations
and build them up: Jeremiah's authority consists entirely in
the word which he transmits to the people. Yahweh sometimes
cautions him to speak his words exactly and precisely, as in the
Temple Sermon: "Speak . . . all the words that I command thee
to speak unto them; diminish not a word" (26:2). Or in Bright's

[4] Isa. 55:1; Wisd. of Sol. 18:5-7; John 7:38-39.
[5] John 4:23; 5:25; etc.
[6] Deut. 18:20; Isa. 6; Jer. 1:4-10; Gal. 1:11-17.

version: "Do not omit a word!"[7] The prophets claim that they repeat Yahweh's judgments to the people; they confront the people with their God. He that rejects the prophet will be judged not by the prophet but by his words, which come from God, so that, in effect, he rejects God when he rejects the words of his messenger (John 12:47-50). Allegorically, writers expressed this conception by identifying the typology of the Day of Yahweh, the Last Judgment, with an analysis of a current historical situation. The prophet speaks to a specific audience at a specific time in history, but the people should see not the prophet but Yahweh. Every choice they make is before God—is eschatological and final. The hour is both coming and now.

In contrast to the classical orator, who finds his authority and his judgment in a particular audience, the prophet has God for his judge and his word as a starting point. If that word differs significantly from the common notions of his society, he cannot change that word in any way. Hence his problem, for God's word by definition is "unheard of." The Suffering Servant confronts the kings with this obstacle. They will shut their mouths, for the prophet will say to them what has never been said before, and they will have to consider what they have never heard before (Isa. 52:15). Or in the famous quotation from Isaiah 55:

> "For my thoughts are not your thoughts,
> Neither are your ways my ways," saith the LORD.
> "For as the heavens are higher than the earth,
> So are my ways higher than your ways,
> And my thoughts than your thoughts."

[8-9]

The prophet tries to span heaven and earth, to bring the one to the other; he can only fail, for who can unite the essentially different? The more clearly he speaks, the less chance he has of bringing his audience into agreement.

The prophet finds himself in a paradoxical situation. God is

7 *Jeremiah*, ed. and trans. John Bright (Garden City, 1965), p. 167.

his authority, for no one will listen to a false prophet; but no one will listen to a true one either. Alienation of an audience is actually a sign of divine inspiration. To the false prophet Hananiah, who prophesied peace to Judah, Jeremiah answered that the earlier prophets never spoke of peace, but of war and ruin.[8] They spoke the baleful and the "unheard of," not what the people desired; so in the Temple Sermon Jeremiah rejected one of the people's most fundamental notions, the belief that no one could ever destroy the Temple.

The people, when they did not react violently to the prophet's word, responded by ignoring it. They honored the prophet but fogot his message. The Jews who killed Gedaliah, the Babylonian governor, carried Jeremiah off with them to Egypt, even though he warned them not to flee there. They obviously did not wish to lose God's prophet, but they simultaneously blocked his words from their minds. The prophets explained this curious mental paralysis metaphorically by calling the people deaf and blind. They have ears and hear not, eyes and see not.[9] They are a foolish people, who listen without understanding; therefore, the word of God becomes a reproach to them, for they can take no delight in it. The prophet responds to this blankness with fury, for he knows that refusal to listen differs little from active resentment. In both cases the people have rejected Yaweh. The prophet speaks to a deaf audience.

The failure of the prophets caused the ruin of their people. In one sense a critic might blame the people for this failure, as Jeremiah does. Through the power of the Lord he claims to know the desperate wickedness of the human heart and its deceitful ways, past all normal comprehension (17:9-10).[10] But

8 Jer. 18:8-9.
9 Ibid., 5:21.
10 In Mark 7:21-23 the heart is described by Jesus as the source of evil; so also in Ps. 95:10-11. This explanation goes back to Egyptian proverbial literature. In the *Instruction of the Vizier Ptah-Hotep* there is the remark: "He whom god loves is a hearkener, [but] he whom god hates cannot hear. It is the heart which brings up its lord as one who hears or as one who does

if the heart is "desperately wicked," who can escape judgment? On the other hand, a critic might blame Yahweh for his "unheard of" messages, which could only upset the people or seem ridiculous. So Isaiah describes his vocation as an active blinding by God of his people:

"Hear ye indeed, but understand not;
And see ye indeed, but perceive not."
Make the heart of this people fat,
And make their ears heavy, and shut their eyes;
Lest they see with their eyes, and hear with their ears,
And understand with their heart, and convert, and be healed.
[6:9-10]

In Mark, Christ spoke in parables *so that* the people might hear and yet misunderstand him.[11] This paradox cannot be explained away. One might argue that the people should never be expected to apprehend the "unheard of," or that they simply refused to listen to new tidings. Both criticisms are true—contradictory or not. For the prophet the situation is intolerable: he speaks for all and against all.

II

The prophet was not the only one who had to struggle with a rhetoric determined by divine inspiration; for in the ancient world, or more particularly in the Roman world, the wise man had to solve much the same problem, whether he was a poet or a philosopher. Like the prophet, the wise man depended upon

---

not hear. The life, prosperity, and health of a man is his heart. . . ." In *Ancient Near Eastern Texts*, ed. James B. Pritchard (Princeton, 1955), p. 414.

[11] This is particularly true in Mark's account. Jesus begins his teaching in the manner of Isaiah. He explains to the Apostles (4:11-12): "Unto you it is given to know the mystery of the kingdom of God: but unto them that are without, all these things are done in parables: that seeing they may see, and not perceive; and hearing they may hear, and not understand; lest at any time they should be converted, and their sins should be forgiven them."

some kind of inspiration, which provided him with the operative control for his discourse, though in his case, the conception of inspiration assumed a more indirect form. The poet and the philosopher devoted themselves to the expression of truth, which generally involved ideas far from the ordinary, even "unheard of" in normal situations. This truth could be anything from the intellectually recondite without any sense of a divine afflatus to a divine truth which included the gods and their manifestations in the cosmos. In the latter situation the inspiration of the wise man approximated that of the prophet, with all the terror and glory that its expression would require. The wise man, however, had one great advantage over the prophet, for he was not constrained to speak out in a specific historical situation. The truth he expressed was a general truth and served the general ends of his society; he did not have to apply a divine dictate to a single political-moral crisis. He could choose his occasion for speech and determine its effects beforehand. To help him in this endeavor he had an acute consciousness of the ordinary man in his possible audience, whom he could not expect to respond to the "unheard of" and whom he could either exclude from his discourse or somehow include on an attenuated basis.

The wise man had three possible ways out of his rhetorical situation, none of which were available to the Hebrew prophet. Two of the ways excluded the multitude completely from truth; the third allowed for a limited participation by the many. In the first the wise man refused to speak out in public and confined himself to conversations with his followers, a method which could be called a form of oral tradition. In the second the wise man wrote down the truth, using a public form of communication, but short-circuiting it, for he made his written discourses unintelligible to the layman. These two ways were generally followed by the philosopher, though the poet at times used the second. Both methods essentially avoid rather than solve the prophet's rhetorical problem, because the wise man never gives the people a chance to know his truth at all. In the third way the wise man resorted to a kind of double talk. Like the prophet he addressed everyone, but he cloaked his truth with myth so that the many, though they might discover the existence of certain things, like the gods and moral rules, could never comprehend them adequately. This was preeminently the way of the poet. He found a model for this rhetoric in the mystery religions, where the hierophant dramatized myths for much the same purposes.

Our own purpose must be, then, to demonstrate first that the poet and the philosopher were conscious of the prophetic dilemma, especially in regard to the many in their audience, and, afterward, to show the three solutions they developed for this problem, beginning with the oral and the written forms of discourse, which were made deliberately unintelligible, and ending with the mythic mode of the poet and hierophant.

The wise men began by rejecting the prophetic paradox. The prophet in his failure had wavered between dismay at the impossible revelations which he received from Yahweh and rage at the blindness of his audience. His blame went in both directions, to God and to the people. The wise man cut this Gordian knot and assigned all the blame to the people, though he remained conscious of the difficulty inherent in the truth he wished to express. Clement of Alexandria argues that the multitude do not judge a speech by the truth but by what pleases them, and what pleases them must be like themselves (*Stromata* 5. 4). Therefore, they cannot receive truth at all, for it is unlike them. Wisdom may go outside and cry out in the streets. She may enter the forum and the marketplace and beg the "simple ones" to leave their simplicity and love knowledge; she may offer to pour out her spirit upon them and explain her words to them. But no matter what she does, they will reject her. She will stretch out her hand in friendship, and no one will regard her (Prov. 1:20-25). Among the late Jewish writers of the Wisdom books, the parabolic visions, and the apocalypses, as well as among many early Christian authors, it was a commonplace that wisdom and truth could not function in the marketplace, an attitude probably created by the failure of the old prophets. Something had to replace prophecy as the vehicle of truth.

Now the sage seeks to avoid wisdom's mistake; knowing ahead of time that most will not heed his call, he stays inside his house and excludes the people from his conversation, either exploiting the symbolic language which Clement claims "is characteristic of the wise man" (*Strom.* 5. 8)[12] or maintaining a public silence. He judges before the event, and quietly damns or ignores the majority of his audience, at least when it comes to speaking seriously about truth. For Clement, Moses' command that the people not approach the Holy Mountain becomes a powerful symbol of this new attitude. Moses necessarily ascended Mount Sinai alone, leaving the multitude far behind and below him, for he was nearing the summit of intellection and contemplation. The dark cloud which covered the mountain signifies "to those capable of understanding" the unbelief and foolishness of the multitude which blocks the light of truth. They do not know that God cannot be expressed in words because he is invisible.[13] Clement is using here the same justification for obscurity that we have already seen in Boccaccio's defense of allegory: "When things perfectly clear seem obscure, it is the beholder's fault" (*GDG* 14. 12). In proverbial language, one may as well talk to a sleeping man as speak the truth to all (Sirach 22:8-9). Worse, such an attempt could destroy the intelligence of the wise:

> Answer not a fool according to his folly,
> Lest thou also be like unto him.
> Answer a fool according to his folly,
> Lest he be wise in his own conceit.
>
> [Prov. 26:4-5]

---

12 The translation is by William Wilson in *The Ante-Nicene Christian Library*, ed. Rev. William Alexander Roberts and James Donaldson (Edinburgh, 1869), vol. 2. Clement is quoting the grammarian Didymus. For a discussion of apocalyptic esotericism, see von Rad, 2: 301-8.

13 *Strom.* 5. 12.

In other words the wise man must not answer the fool at all; no communication is best. Silence is preferable even to allegory. Philosophers like Ammonius Saccas, the teacher of Plotinus and Origen, felt constrained to maintain a public silence, as Pico says in the *Heptaplus* of another philosopher: "Pythagoras became a master of silence, and he himself did not entrust anything to writing except a very few things which, when dying, he left to his daughter Dama" (Pro. 1).[14]

The wise man, when possible, avoided all forms of writing, since written documents could be read by anyone, and confined himself to oral instruction given to a few followers; this is much like the picture John draws of Christ at the Last Supper, verbally explaining his revelation to his Apostles and preparing them for his death and resurrection. Pico, on the authority of Dionysius the Areopagite, argues that the early Christians likewise shielded their truth by oral instruction. It was their custom never to commit their more secret doctrines to writing but to rely upon the spoken word and to communicate their secrets only to an inner circle of initiates (*Hep.* Pro. 1).[15] Oral tradition guarded the sanctuary of truth, for the Hebrews as well as for the Greeks and Christians, as Clement thinks: "For there were certainly, among the Hebrews, some things delivered unwritten" (*Strom.* 5. 10). Moses reserved the understanding of the Law for oral discourse. He proclaimed the Law to all the people and placed it in the Ark of Covenant, but he never wrote down its interpretation, which he revealed orally, "under a great holy seal of silence," to Joshua and later to the high priests (Pico, *On the Dignity*). The last hierophant of Eleusis carried with him to his grave the secrets of the Mysteries, handed down orally for end-

[14] Porphyry *On the Life of Plotinus* 3. The translation from Pico is by Douglas Carmichael in *Pico della Mirandola* (Indianapolis, 1965), hereafter referred to as *PdM*. The phrase appears on p. 172 of Eugenio Garin's edition of *De hominis dignitate, Heptaplus, De ente et uno* (Florence, 1942), hereafter referred to as Garin.

[15] Origen makes the same point. See *Periarchon* 4. 2. 4.

less ages, and never since discovered by all the efforts of scholarship and archeology.[16]

Ultimately, the philosopher, unlike the hierophant, had to break his public silence, try as he might to avoid doing it; for he could never communicate with anyone outside his small coterie of immediate disciples if he relied solely on oral instruction. Porphyry's story in his *Life of Plotinus* well illustrates this dilemma. Three disciples of Ammonius Saccas—Erennius, Origen, and Plotinus—had agreed among themselves not to reveal the ideas of their master to anyone. Plotinus remained true to this agreement, never relating anything of Ammonius' system even in his unpublished lectures, but the other two eventually broke the compact. Erennius first began to write up the philosophic positions of Ammonius, and then Origen put out two treatises: *On the Spirit-Beings* and, in Gallienus' reign, *The King the Sole Creator*. Plotinus still held back, though he began to base his lectures on the ideas of his master, but by the first year of the reign of Gallienus, Plotinus too had begun to write (*Life* 3). The conspiracy of silence could not last.

But if the wise man must finally speak out, he can still avoid the prophetic dilemma by adopting the second mode of exclusive rhetoric: he can write in a fashion absolutely unintelligible to the many. The writer of *Horapollo* defines the objectives of this rhetorical mode in figurative terms. The word of truth can be compared to dew falling by night on plants and stones. The plants receive the dew and grow, but on the rocks the dew evaporates. Now the wise man must alter the natural order and see to it that the dew falls solely on plants (1. 37)—a seemingly impossible objective, but not really so difficult outside the metaphoric description. The Hermetic writers describe the standard solution to this situation, though with their own terminology and outlook. They say that God offered Mind to all men but

[16] For Pico the translation is by C. G. Wallis in *PdM*. In Garin, p. 154. For Eleusis, see Mylonas, p. 281.

that not everyone accepted the gift. Those who did could perceive the Good and could realize that existence in the sensible world was a misfortune for them. Those who ignored the offer, on the other hand, continued to live a life devoted to the things of sense and could not "admire the things that are worthy of contemplation."[17] Now everyone, both fools and wise men, shares the gift of speech, but only the wise have Mind. Therefore, the Hermetic rhetorician could create a Mind-speech, incomprehensible to the many, since they could not possibly understand the "unheard of." In short, the wise man needs to develop a private language, open only to those familiar with his terminology. This was the method common among philosophers. Aristotle is said to have remarked that his treatises on divine matters were both written and not written. He meant that they were intelligible only to his disciples. Someone who casually picked up a tract of Plotinus would not read very far. The philosopher automatically made the dew of his words fall where he wanted it to fall . . . on the intellectual elite.

On occasion, the mystagogue and the poet also practiced this mode of rhetoric, though in their own fashion. The priests of Isis wrote out the sacred formulas of initiation in hieroglyphic script or in illegible characters (*Golden Ass* 11. 48), a crude method but none the less effective. The later poets and prophets in the Jewish tradition found more sophisticated forms of this obscurantism in parable and apocalyptic vision, made absolutely dark and confusing for those who could not break the cipher.[18] Christ tells his disciples in Mark that he can explain to them orally the mystery of God's kingdom but that to others he must speak in parables, for the reasons given by Isaiah. They must see and not perceive, hear and not understand, lest they should

[17] *Hermetica* 4. 5, translated by Robert Grant in *Gnosticism* (New York, 1961). The following anecdote about Aristotle comes from Aulus Gellius *Noct. Att.* 20. 5 and is repeated by Reynolds in *Mythomystes*. See Spingarn, 1: 157.

[18] The metaphor is in von Rad, 2: 302.

repent at any time and their sins be forgiven (4:10-12).[19] Explanations of the parables are reserved for the initiate.

Both these rhetorical modes, the oral and the written, avoided rather than solved the prophetic dilemma. The philosopher simply excluded the multitude from his discourse; he never spoke to them at all. Only the poet and the priest, through their allegorical myths, provided some sort of direct solution to the prophetic problem. They discovered a way to accommodate the multitude by their rhetoric, while they simultaneously communicated truth to the elite.

To understand the manner in which the allegorical poet and the hierophant spanned heaven and earth and yet succeeded where the prophet failed, we must first clarify the precise objectives of this third rhetorical mode and then examine the role played by the many and the few within it. We will see that the allegorist did not permanently divide his audience into two parts, but left a small door open through which some of the multitude could join the ranks of the elite. Finally, we will show what key the allegorist gave to the few, by which they could unlock the secrets of his myths, that key being a common theory of the cosmos.

The allegorist had for his end the same general objectives which the prophet had: the moral reform of the multitude and the proclamation of truth; but he achieved these ends by means which the prophet could not accept. He separated truth from morality, the "unheard of" from its practical manifestations. Outside the Judeo-Christian tradition, this separation created what in prophetic terms would be called idol worship. Although the initiates in the *Asclepius* worshipped the One, the other

19 I do not quarrel with those who argue about the so-called Messianic secret and provide a political justification for the parabolic rhetoric of the Gospels, though I do consider such explanations superficial. They do not take into account the prophet's rhetorical dilemma, nor do they represent a Renaissance understanding of the situation. My explanation corresponds to that of Pico, who himself knew and understood the late classical theories of obscurantist rhetoric.

Egyptians honored numerous gods. Likewise, the elite within Mithraism knew the Iranian myths, whereas the others studied Chaldean astrology.[20] The worship of the crocodile or the ibis might well control the moral customs of the Egyptians, but the Hebrew prophet could never accept the price of this reformation. It meant that the allegorist disguised by his myths a logical contradiction; he could not assert simultaneously that there are many gods and that there is only one god or, in Mithraism, that man must choose between good and evil and that man's destiny is completely determined by the stars. The allegorist could defend his practice, however, and contend that his myth disguised a paradox, that is, a contradiction open to explanation. He could argue that most of his audience only had the capacity to see many gods, while a few could see better, even to the One behind the Many. What the initiate knew as paradox could only exist as contradiction for the multitude, if they had everything told to them at once. Hence, concealment. He could further argue that the many simply could not bear a direct presentation of truth. The Hebrews gathered around Mount Sinai recoiled in fear from the thunder and lightning of Yahweh's voice and asked for a mediator. The allegorist put himself in the role of this mediator, reserving the terrors of the "unheard of" for the few who could bear it.

The sort of moral control which the allegorist exercised over the multitude varied from the rudimentary to a complete code of behavior. The votaries of Cybele, who took part in the spring celebrations of their goddess, received from the ritual little more than a knowledge that the gods exist. They did not know the nature of the gods, experiencing them, rather, in the way in which they perceived the objects of the sense world—without understanding.[21] They heard the proclamation and learned that

[20] Frances Yates, *Giordano Bruno and the Hermetic Tradition* (Chicago, 1964), p. 142, hereafter referred to as *GB*; and Franz Cumont, *The Mysteries of Mithra* (New York, 1956), pp. 119-20.

[21] Sallustius, *Concerning the Gods and the Universe*, ed. A. D. Nock (Cambridge, 1926), iii.

the gods do affect their lives, but without adequate comprehension. How could the women who witnessed the mythic drama of Attis and the Great Mother possibly have known that the tale really explained in allegorical terms generation in the material cosmos? Yet the Emperor Julian thought such a limited understanding adequate:[22]

> Now I think ordinary men derive benefit enough from the irrational myth which instructs them through symbols alone. But those who are more highly endowed with wisdom will find the truth about the gods helpful. . . .
>
> [*Oration* 5. 170b]

They actually learned more than bare facts; they discovered something of the history of the gods. Onatas the Neopythagorean remarks: "So God is Himself neither visible nor perceptible, but rather is to be contemplated only by reason and mind. But His works and deeds are clearly perceptible to all men."[23] Knowledge of divine action can lead to a more complete morality. As Origen argues, a literal understanding of revelation will edify the multitude and exercise a moral control over their lives (*Periarchon* 4. 2. 5-6), an idea Pico della Mirandola develops in his well-known *Oration*, when he says that Moses announced the Law for the moral benefit of all Israel, though restricting its understanding to Joshua and the chief priests, who interpreted it allegorically.[24] Now the Law governed every action in a man's life. Thus, the allegorist could affect in some cases the entire moral code of a people.

More important, the allegorist, in contrast to the philosopher, did not permanently exclude the many from truth, for he recognized that a few of them could pass over into the elite, sometimes through a whole series of stages. The prophet never had this possibility open to him, because he had revealed truth to

[22] In the Loeb translation.

[23] Quoted by Erwin Goodenough, *By Light, Light* (New Haven, 1935), p. 20. The Greek in parentheses is omitted.

[24] Reynolds quotes another such passage from Pico. See Spingarn, 1: 161.

the many once and for all and they had rejected it. The multitude in the audience of the allegorist did not encounter truth in so uncompromising a manner. Since it was concealed from them, at least initially, they could gradually move closer and closer to it. As in the Renaissance, various divisions could be applied to this audience, according to the number of interpretations possible for a given allegory. Origen classifies the Christians into three groups: body, soul, and spirit. The literal story aids those who have not yet transcended "body"; the moral, those in whom "soul" is dominant; the spiritual, those who have reached the ultimate stage of development.[25] The divisions correspond to a common Hellenistic theory of the tripartite soul. In the Mysteries of Eleusis an individual went through three stages of initiation,[26] but the number could be still larger. The worshipers of Mithras had seven, all with distinctive dress and names: the Raven, the Nymphus or Bride, the Soldier, the Lion, the Persian, the Heliodromus or Courier of the Sun, and highest, the Father, who wore a red tunic and mantle, a broad yellow girdle, and a red Phrygian cap.[27] The Roman Catholic ritual still preserves these grades of initiation. To become a priest one must go through seven orders: tonsure, door-keeper, lector, exorcist, acolyte, subdeacon, and deacon, each one of which has different assigned functions and dress.

The criteria for passing over from the many to the few varied from one writer to another, but the same general attitude predominated. Origen asked for moral qualities: chastity, sobriety, and watchfulness (*Peri.* 4. 2. 7); Augustine for more: charity, purity of heart, a good conscience, and an unfeigned faith (*De doctrina* 1. 40. 44).[28] Sallustius sounds more like a Renaissance theorist. He wants the members of his elite to have had a good

---

[25] *Peri.* 4. 2. 4.

[26] Mylonas, p. 239.

[27] M. J. Vermaseren and C. C. Van Essen, *Excavations in the Mithraeum of the Church of Santa Prisca in Rome* (Leiden, 1965), pp. 155-60.

[28] Origen's list exists in Rufinus' translation.

education, all the way from childhood, free from an environment where foolish ideas are tolerated. They must have a good and intelligent nature, without which education would be of no use, since the individual must share an essential likeness with the gods he wishes to find (*Concerning the Gods* 1). In all these writers it is assumed that the seeker for truth must first make himself like it in some way, before he can ever hope to recognize truth when he sees it. In Platonic terms, only he who possesses a beautiful soul can see Intelligible Beauty.

Anyone could try to pass the gulf separating the initiate from the uninitiate, but few ever made the transition. Reynolds quotes Pico to this effect in *Mythomystes*. In the ascent to truth the individual must first recognize through philosophical study that sensible beauty by itself cannot suffice, that it represents a higher beauty beyond sense. Second, the individual must persevere in his efforts and maintain a proper elevation of mind, otherwise he will never be ravished in ecstasy beyond the earth. Everyone can participate in this celestial love, but few actually do (Spingarn, 1: 151). Most people cannot maintain the proper elevation of mind, nor can they wholly reject sensible beauty. Even among the Christians the few would be limited because, though salvation was offered to all, its understanding re-created the ironic situation of the Hebrew prophet. Few people could be expected to respond much more than superficially to the "unheard of." To quote a modern presentation of the dilemma:[29]

The difference between a genius and a Christian is that a genius is nature's extraordinary, no man being able to make himself a genius, whereas a Christian is freedom's extraordinary, or, more properly, freedom's ordinary, for though it is found extraordinarily seldom, it is what everyone ought to be. Therefore God wills that Christianity should be preached to all men absolutely, therefore the Apostles are very simple men, and the Pattern is in the lowly form of a servant, all this in order to indicate that this extraordinary is the ordinary,

[29] The Kierkegaard translation is by Walter Lowrie (Boston, 1956), p. 159.

is accessible to all—but for all that a Christian is a thing even more rare than a genius.

[Kierkegaard, *Attack upon "Christendom"*]

Whether one establishes philosophical or religious criteria, whether one looks like Sallustius to those of natural talents or tries like Pico to revive the spark hidden in all men, the result is much the same. Few really know the truth, because few really want it. Mankind cannot bear too much reality.

One might well ask then how the allegorist expects anyone to penetrate his mysteries at all. His own critical metaphors, that of the cloud and that of the veil, further emphasize his difficulties in this respect because they are drawn from particular historical situations where only one person managed to make the full transition. Clement identified the image of the cloud with the revelation on Mount Sinai. At that time Moses alone was allowed to climb the mountain and enter the dark cloud where God was. Some others—Joshua, Aaron, Nadab, Abihu, and seventy elders—were able to approach the cloud, but all the other Israelites had to remain far off and could not even touch the mountain on pain of death.[30] The veil image pointed to the same idea. It was based on the structure and ceremony of the Jerusalem Temple or Moses' Tabernacle; it covered the Holy of Holies. No one passed through this veil except the High Priest once a year—surely an extreme reduction of the few! Outside, the people ranged in increasing numbers as their distance from the Holy of Holies increased, ending finally with the gentiles, confined to the outer court.[31] Likewise at Eleusis, though the initiates could enter the temenos of Demeter, only the Hierophant could go into the Anaktoron, where the holy objects were kept.[32]

The poet and the priest viewed this problem of the elite in differing perspectives, which taken together represented the old

[30] *Strom.* 5. 12.
[31] Heb. 9:1-7; *Strom.* 5. 6; Goodenough, pp. 96-98.
[32] Mylonas, p. 236.

prophetic dilemma—the "unheard of." The prophet had presented truth to the people which they could not understand, a function much like that of the allegorical poet; but at the same time he confronted the people with superhuman power, something which the priest usually did. The hierophant had to guard his mysteries carefully because the safety of his people and sometimes the whole world depended on his care. For Iamblichus the cosmic order of things remains stable: "because the ineffable arcane in Abydos [or in the inner shrine] are never at any time revealed to profane contemplation" (*Mysteries* 14).[33] The priest himself faced extreme danger when he invoked the gods, for he was calling upon active beings which far surpassed him in knowledge and strength. In the *Heptaplus* Pico remarks that the angels enjoy "eternal life and unchanging activity" (*Hep.* Pro. 2); they are a permanent, active power. Myth had such power because it put mankind into communication with the greater forces in the cosmos. Iamblichus describes the terrifying situation of the priest, calling upon a deity, but taking precautions, for he cannot be certain that other deities will not also respond to his prayer. The words and symbols of truth had magical potency and could bring about the destruction of someone who used them illicitly.[34] Apuleius has the High Priest of Isis say to Lucius that no votary of the goddess ever dared to participate in her mysteries without her express permission. To do so would be sacrilegious; it would be an attempt at self-destruction. Isis holds in her power the gates of the underworld and the principle of life, and the initiate goes through a voluntary death, hoping precariously for a resurrection into life. The penalty for sacrilege at Eleusis was death.[35] The rending of the veil over the Jewish Sanctuary meant catastrophe for man's physical and moral worlds. Pico so describes the effects of the Crucifixion. At Christ's death the veil of the Temple was rent in two, exposing to view the room where the

33 The translation is by Alexander Wilder (Greenwich, 1915), p. 235.
34 *Mysteries* 13; Garin, p. 184.
35 *Golden Ass* 11. 48; Mylonas, pp. 225-26.

angels dwelt. His death broke the barriers between the sublunary and the supercelestial worlds and bore all the signs of an
apocalypse: earthquakes, preternatural gloom, the darkened sun,
and the resurrection of the dead.[36] The rending of the veil meant
something like an apocalypse, because it signified the breaking
forth of enormous power into the world of men, power beyond
all human control and capable of both good and evil. Now the
prophet necessarily rent this veil every time he spoke; he broke
down the defenses of the hierophant and confronted the people
directly with the divine power. The result was apocalypse.

The poet viewed the problem of the elite in terms of communication. Like the prophet he served his inspiration and had
to express the "unheard of," and for the poet this incomprehensible truth manifested itself in the veil of allegory. He could not
avoid speaking in obscure language, even if he wished, because
the nature of the truth he had to express demanded it. The
prophet had only to transmit specific directives, however impossible, but the poet had to reveal the nature of the unknown itself.
He was concerned with presenting physical and psychic truths:
the actions of the gods in the cosmos and their power within
man's soul (*Concerning the Gods* 4). But the gods, being themselves invisible and beyond human thought, could not be expressed in simple speech, so myths had to become enigmatic and
obscure, if the poet wanted to remain faithful to his inspiration.[37]
They were in a sense his gifts to the gods, and one must make a
gift suitable to its recipient. A father does not give his five-year-
old child a copy of Wittgenstein. Likewise, in a rhetorical situation a speaker must keep proper decorum. He does not address
Queen Elizabeth in the same terms he would use for a class of
school children or for a labor rally. Myths too, since they are
addressed unto the gods, must be like to the nature of the gods

---

[36] *Hep*. Pro. 2, p. 188 in Garin.

[37] Clement goes further. In *Strom*. 5. 10 he says, "For the God of the
universe, who is above all speech, all conception, all thought, can never be
committed to writing, being inexpressible even by His own power."

in order to please them. Since the gods surpass man in power and wisdom, the myth must represent both what man can say about them and what he cannot say. It must include both the obvious and the obscure. All the inspired poets, the greatest philosophers, and the founders of religious observances employed the dark speech which the gods themselves used when they spoke to man through oracles (*Concerning the Gods* 3). Obscurity or depth signifies the presence of the gods and likewise demonstrates that the poet or myth-maker participates in divinity. Like the prophet, he justifies his noncommunication with the people by the divinity which inspires him. The gods, not the people, exercise the real control over allegory; they themselves determine its nature. Now, though unintelligible language might please the gods,[38] it did not help the poet communicate with even the elite. He had to find a way to help them, so that they could interpret his myths rightly.

He found an answer to his rhetorical problem in his own subject matter. If the poet expresses the actions of the gods in the cosmos and in the human soul, he can at least assume that the educated elite will share the same general theory about the universe and the soul; namely, that the soul mirrors the universe as microcosm to macrocosm. It follows then that a *single* theory of the cosmos will serve to explicate the poet's allegories, even on the psychic level, and restrict the kinds of interpretation possible to any given myth. The poet's allegories can serve as a true and precise mode of communication between the few. Modern critics find a similar control for themselves in anthropology and psychology. They too could find in myth a depth and suggestiveness, but they could never achieve quite the particularity and detail in depth which a Sallustius had because they must choose between many conflicting theories and do not have such a common and concrete theory shared by all. They could not speak out mythically in public like the wise man or poet of old and expect

[38] *Mysteries* 15. Iamblichus is actually defending the use of foreign terms in the mysteries, but the principle extends logically to allegorical myth.

such a consensus in detailed understanding as the ancients could expect, for the ancients had in the cosmos a key to unlock the sanctuary of the mysteries.

The elite audience will assume that the poet is exploiting in his allegorical myths the interrelationship of the three worlds which make up the universe: the supercelestial, the celestial, and the sublunary. They will recognize in poetic myth a form of depth discourse, in which the poet talks about many things at the same time, using an image in one world to signify its corollaries in the other two. This is a position assumed by Julian and Sallustius and later by Pico in his Second Proem to the *Heptaplus*. The poet can apply celestial or earthly symbols to divine things, which can be represented as stars, wheels, animals, or one of the elements. Likewise, divine names can signify earthly things. The poet moves up and down the chain of concord, literally exchanging natures as well as names among the three orders. He practices allegory, speaking in a symbolic fashion which he bases not on his subjective imagination but on the objective order of the universe.[39]

Critics see the principle of cosmic exegesis behind even the standard metaphors used to characterize the nature of allegorical myth itself. For example, in the sphinx image, which Pico and Plutarch base upon the Egyptian practice of placing human-headed animals before their temples (*Hep.* Pro. 1; *Isis and Osiris* 9), Clement understands both the "enigmatical and obscure" doctrine respecting God and the "harmony of the world" (*Strom.* 5. 5, 8). Likewise, the veil image was interpreted in cosmic fashion. For Philo the veil separated the Holy of Holies from the Sanctuary, or, in allegorical terms, the Invisible from the Visible world, the Powers from the Cosmos.[40] Clement identified the veil instead with the outer veil of the Temple but with much the same meaning. It divided the worlds of intellect and sense,

[39] *Hep.* Pro. 2, pp. 190-92 in Garin.
[40] Goodenough, p. 113. Philo would also agree with Clement's understanding of the outer veil.

separating the altar of incense from popular unbelief (*Strom.* 5. 6). Pico developed a Philonian interpretation. Men and animals could enter the outermost part of the tabernacle; so it symbolized the lowest of the three worlds. The Sanctuary with its shining gold and seven-branched candlestick signified the celestial world with the seven planets. The Holy of Holies, which contained the ark shadowed by the cherubim, obviously stood for the supercelestial world.[41]

A discussion of one or two myths might help to clarify these principles of cosmic interpretation. Sallustius explicates two ritual myths: the judgment of Paris and the mutilation of Attis.[42] In the former story Strife or Discord throws a golden apple amid the gods at one of their banquets, and Hera, Athena, and Aphrodite contend for it. Zeus has Paris arbitrate the dispute, and he gives the apple to Aphrodite. Sallustius argues that the banquet symbolizes the supercelestial powers of the gods, gathered into consort. The golden apple is the universe, for it is thrown by Strife and the cosmos is made up of opposites. The gods fight for the apple; that is, they give various gifts to the cosmos. Paris assigns the apple to Aphrodite because, existing as he does in the world of sense, the only higher power which he can see is the beauty which informs material bodies.

The second of Sallustius' myths, that of Attis, was one of the most important ritual myths in antiquity, performed every spring by the worshipers of the Great Mother. In the story Cybele finds Attis by the river Gallus, falls in love with him, and gives him her cap of stars. Attis betrays her with a nymph, and the Mother in revenge drives him mad so that he castrates himself, leaves the nymph, and returns to her. A savage tale, but Sallustius manages to make of it a cosmic theology. Cybele represents the principle of life; Attis, the demiurge who made the world of becoming. The Mother of the Gods finds him by the river Gallus, which symbolizes the Milky Way (Galaxias Kyklos), which divides the

41 *Hep.* Pro. 2, pp. 186-88 in Garin.
42 *Concerning the Gods* 4.

world of change from the supercelestial world. The Mother loves Attis and gives him power, signified by the starry cap, for the supercelestial powers love the celestial. Attis loves the nymph, who presides over becoming, since her element, water, indicates flux. Attis' castration demonstrates that cosmic generation cannot go on endlessly, lest inferior existence give birth to still lower forms of being. Thus, he casts away his generative organs and returns to the gods, from whom he came. The Emperor Julian gives a fuller explication of this myth in his *Fifth Oration*, but he differs in no essentials from Sallustius, except, perhaps, when he makes the nymph the cause set over matter. In both Julian and Sallustius the story is read in the same cosmic terms.

The cosmos, then, solved for the poet the most difficult part of the prophet's dilemma. Assuming a common theory of the universe, the poet could safely cloak his truth with myth and expect the educated few to perceive his "unheard of" revelation through the veils of allegory. He could simultaneously affect the morals of the multitude and create gnosis among the few. He did all that the prophet had tried to do by separating the two aspects of the prophetic mission: his revelation of truth and his desire for moral reform. The prophet had attempted to stimulate moral improvement directly by the truth he had received from God, and the result was failure. The allegorist, dividing truth from morality by the veil of myth, achieved both ends—at least in theory. The people learned morality from the story of the poet, and the wise understood it.

The poet could succeed where the prophet failed because he had a somewhat different purpose for his rhetoric. The prophet spoke on specific occasions and wanted to remedy a particular situation, while the poet wished to serve the permanent end of his society—union with the gods. Plutarch remarks in his treatise, *On Isis and Osiris:* "The fact is that nothing of man's usual possessions is more divine than reasoning [speech], especially reasoning about the gods; and nothing has a greater influence toward happiness . . ." (68).[43] The poet revealed divine truth to his society, telling it in story form, with a before and after. In a sense he rationalized unchanging truth, converting the eternal into the temporal medium of speech; hence, the story form. The simultaneous became sequential, though in the interpretation the before and after disappeared.[44] Within his stories the poet placed man in a divine context in which he could discover his proper attributes by comparison with the higher beings in the cosmos. He gave profundity to the human situation by creating an objective vertical dimension, where man found himself on a ladder with other beings above and below him. His allegorical myths were necessary to the very life of society, mirroring it in a magical fashion which at the same time revealed value—the invisible standards by which man lives in the visible cosmos, once he realizes his own nature.

It is for these reasons, perhaps, that the ancients attributed religion itself to the poets. Homer established the personalities and described the rituals of the Olympian gods, and Orpheus reformed the Bacchic mysteries, acting as both priest and poet. His allegorical myths determined the Orphic rituals; his poetry preceded his religion.[45] With such ideas in mind, Hermes Trismegistus argues in the *Asclepius* that literally all religions follow from poetic myth. The supreme divinity sent the Muses to man to teach him religion by their inspired song (9), an idea which Puttenham repeats in the Renaissance. The poets first performed sacrifices to the gods with invocations and sacred rituals. They invented religion with all its observances and ceremonies and became its first priests and ministers (*Arte* 1. 3). They created the moral values of society and revealed to man the divine.

Nevertheless, the figure of the allegorical poet cannot quite

[43] In the Loeb translation.

[44] Contained in the comments following Sallustius' discussion of the Attis myth (*Concerning the Gods* 4), pp. 8-9 in Nock.

[45] W. K. C. Guthrie contends that Orphism was a religion based upon the written word. See *Orpheus and Greek Religion* (New York, 1966), p. 69.

make sense, particularly to modern critics, without a knowledge of the corresponding figure of the prophet. Not only does the prophet show how a similar rhetorical problem can be treated in another fashion, but, more especially, he justifies the obscurantism of the allegorist. Without a knowledge of the prophetic dilemma and failure, a critic cannot really appreciate the allegorist's frantic concern with concealment, with his mythic veil. He cannot understand why the poet thought that he had to hide his truth, unless he already knows all the problems this truth can cause both for the speaker and for his audience. The allegorist seldom explained why he had to conceal his truth; he simply assumed it. That is why the defenses of allegory, like that of Boccaccio, sound arbitrary and unfair to modern sensibilities, when read alone. The allegorist does not explain enough about what he is doing, but the figure of the prophet provides the needed commentary.

Most of the writers on allegory whom we have discussed in this chapter came from the same milieu—that of late classical antiquity, which itself influenced so much of Renaissance "classicism." Clement, Philo, and Origen all came from Alexandria, the seedbed of Neoplatonism in the early centuries of the Empire; Sallustius and Julian came later, being part of the pagan revival in the mid-fourth century. They share a basically common attitude toward allegory, particularly in their emphasis on cosmic exegesis, the mode of communication among the wise. In the Renaissance the Florentine Platonists revived their ideas, though they never really died even in the Middle Ages. Pico made the theory of the cosmos the primary means of his allegorical interpretation and based much of his theory of human nature on the microcosm and macrocosm. Edmund Spenser practiced a form of cosmic allegory all his life, from *The Shepheardes Calender* to the Mutabalitie Cantos, but he need not have read the Florentines to find this approach to allegory. He could have found analogous ideas in Plutarch's *Isis and Osiris* or in Golding's Ovid. It is with these late classical principles in mind that we must study the specifically Renaissance theories of allegory. At the same time we must try to experience within ourselves something of the excitement which allegorical rhetoric could give to the ancient world and to the Renaissance. It was not a process of mere interpretation, such as we practice in our schools today; it was a revelation. Who can say what it must have been like to discover through story one's own nature, the universe, and the invisible powers? Apuleius has a description of the experience, which must have been as absolute and shattering as death:[46]

> I approached neere unto Hell, even to the gates of Proserpina, and after that, I was ravished throughout all the Element, I returned to my proper place: About midnight I saw the Sun shine, I saw likewise the gods celestiall and gods infernall, before whom I presented my selfe, and worshipped them. . . .
>
> [*Golden Ass* 11.48]

[46] In the translation by William Aldington, which was popular during the period. I am using a modern reprint (London, 1930).

❧ 3 ❧

The Theory of Allegory

So far we have been concerned with distinguishing allegory from other forms of rhetoric; and, in the course of this investigation, we have had time only for brief sketches of its theory and background. In the next section of this book we can concentrate solely on allegory itself: its theory, its rhetorical function, its interpretation and practice. A basic motif running through much of this discussion will be the oral character of allegorical art, an idea to which we will return again and again. The term *allegory* itself and its cognates make no sense in a written context, for they invariably presuppose some kind of judgment by an auditor; and a modern critic finds it quite impossible to understand the function of allegory in a society, which was largely memorial, without recourse to oral poetry. We know that ancient society found in Homer's epics a kind of memory bank, but we seldom think of *The Faerie Queene* in these terms because we draw sharp differences between what we regard as true oral poetry, dependent as it is on oral formulas, and poetry which, though written to be read aloud, does not depend on such formulaic techniques. The Renaissance poet like Spenser, however, was not himself conscious of these differences and, consequently, evaluated his own rhetorical role in terms half-alien to those of a modern critic of the period. As a result, we ourselves have become blind to another set of differences, those which separate our own theories of allegory from those current in the Renaissance.

The educated people of the Renaissance generally used the term *allegory* in one of three ways. In its narrowest sense they

54

applied it to a particular figure of speech, one of the tropes of sentences; that is, a figure which requires interpretation by an auditor and does not simply create a sound pattern in the ear. Unlike a metaphor, which is also a trope, a sentence trope depends for its existence upon two or more words (a "sentence"). In a wider sense they sometimes equated allegory with all the tropes of sentences, in which meaning allegory defined all extended tropological discourse. Both these uses of the term come from the rhetorical handbooks. The third application of the word belonged to the critics of poetry, who took the term from the rhetoricians and used it to define poetry itself, which they envisaged as extended tropological discourse. Thus, to understand its meaning in poetics we must begin with the rhetorical manuals.

Everyone is familiar with the old definition of allegory as a single trope. It can be called a continued metaphor or a "forme of speech which expresseth one thing in words, and another in sense."[1] The poverty of language in part necessitates this figure, for there are many things for which no words exist. To refer to them a speaker resorts to analogy, signifying an unnamable B by an A which has a name. Generally this consists in applying the names of external objects or physical experiences to the invisible aspects of human passion, thought, or action.[2] But in a wider sense allegory depends upon the wealth of language as well as upon its poverty. Language has many words for one thing as well as things for which it has no words. Ralph Lever in the Preface to his *Arte of Reason* makes of this fact a formula: many words can have the same meaning and one word can have several

---

[1] Peacham, *The Garden of Eloqvence* (London, 1593), p. 25.

[2] Tasso in his *Account of the Allegory* in *Jerusalem Delivered* argues in this sense. He claims that allegory represents the hidden aspect of passions, opinions, and customs. It expresses the inward as opposed to the outward side of things, for which men have analogical language derivative from the names for objects of sense. See Henry Morley's edition of the Fairfax translation (London, 1890), p. 436.

meanings.[3] Spenser exploits this double principle in his developed
allegories, where Belphoebe, Gloriana, and Mercilla all refer to
Queen Elizabeth, while, at the same time, Gloriana signifies two
things: the Queen and glory itself. A diagram might help to
clarify this matter:

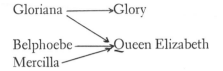

And, of course, both Belphoebe and Mercilla signify things other
than the English Queen. The principle may seem difficult in
theory and is certainly complex in practice (one could never
really diagram the allegory of *The Faerie Queene*), but it depends upon the habitual operation of language and is as old as
man himself.

In his *Garden of Eloqvence* (1593) Peacham notes an important corollary of this principle when he says that not all the
words in an allegory have a transposed meaning. Some of them
preserve their normal signification within an allegorical context.
For his example, Peacham uses an allegory of ambition, where
the foolish attempt of the rustic to pluck the fruit on the "top
of the topmost branch" describes by analogy the dangerous activity of the ambitious man. In his exhortation to this type of person, the speaker uses the words *couet, consider,* and *forethinke*
in their ordinary sense:[4]

> Why doest thou *couet* the frute, and not *consider* the height
> of the tree whereon it groweth? thou doest not *forethinke* of
> the difficultie in climbing, nor danger in reaching, wherby
> it cometh to passe, that while thou endeuorest to climbe to

[3] In a passage quoted by R. F. Jones, *The Triumph of the English Language* (Stanford, 1953), p. 126.

[4] The earlier phrase is Sappho's in the Lattimore translation. See the
eighth selection in *Greek Lyrics* (Chicago, 1961). For Peacham, see the
Garden, pp. 26-27. The italics are mine.

the top, thou fallest with the bough which thou doest embrace.

Similarly, the details within an allegorical scene need not all have transposed significance. Some of them merely set the scene. The flowers which the nymphs strew at the foot of Arlo Hill are real flowers and help to establish the setting of Nature's judgment of Mutabilitie (*FQ* 7. 7. 10). Through the presence of Nature they may take on an added meaning, but they never lose their proper significance.

It is the critic's function to fill in the unspoken part of the analogy when he examines an allegory. As Rosemond Tuve has demonstrated, metaphoric discourse is open-ended; it demands interpretation, and often the critic will find more than one interpretation which can fit.[5] Peacham's story about the fruit-picker could as well describe the Pelagian, who thinks that he can save himself by his own efforts. Some control in this criticism is provided by a proper attention to the way in which Renaissance poets habitually used the "places" from which they derived their analogies. Peacham, for example, in his discussion of metaphor remarks that mental operations are generally represented in visual terms and affections of the heart by aural images. The Red Cross Knight perceives the Heavenly Jerusalem with its walls of pearl and Angels' Tower exclusively by means of vision (1. 10. 55-58). Likewise, Duessa appears in striking visual images (for example, clad in scarlet with a Persian mitre [1. 2. 13]), for she symbolizes error or wandering from truth. Guyon, on the other hand (in the Bower of Bliss) is beset by a combination of aural and visual temptations. As he approaches Acrasia and Verdant, he hears a wondrous symphony, where "consorted in one harmonee,/Birdes, voyces, instruments, windes, waters, all agree" (2. 12. 70), and then someone chants the famous Song of the Rose. Guyon's problem involves more of the affections of the heart than does that of the Red Cross Knight. Similar observa-

[5] Tuve, *Allegorical Imagery* (Princeton, 1966), p. 220.

tions can be made of the other senses and "places." Smell, for example, can indicate foresight, since a person often perceives the presence of an object by its odor before he sees it. One "smells out" a conspiracy before the evidence can be found. This list of "places" could be expanded indefinitely, but these examples suffice to show that the auditor had certain habitual guidelines to follow when he filled in the open-end of the poet's allegory.

In its first sense, then, allegory can be described as a figure of speech incomplete in itself, which, for this very reason, makes certain demands on an audience. The hearer by analogy must fill in the proper meaning to complete the figure. It follows that allegorical figures presuppose a certain cooperation between a speaker and an auditor; the former makes a statement and the latter completes it by his interpretation.

In its second sense allegory could be used as a descriptive term for all the tropes of sentences. Sherry simply calls allegory the "seconde parte of Trope."[6] As such, all the related tropes like irony and proverb formed its subspecies. This identification was possible because allegory had the same loose definition as that given to the whole class of tropes: one thing in word, another in meaning. This definition itself rests upon an old classical theory of oral discourse. Tertullian distinguishes two kinds of words: the *sermo* and the *ratio* or idea (*Apologeticus* 21. 10), a division which corresponds to the old Stoic classification of *lógos* as *'endiáthetos* (in the mind) and *prophorikós* (uttered or spoken).[7] There is the word in the mind and the spoken word; when these two differ, we are in tropological discourse. The auditor forms within himself a different word from the one he hears. Sometimes this unspoken word closely resembles its aural counterpart; sometimes it hardly resembles the spoken word at all. The various tropes of sentences differ from each other according to the degree in which the *lógos prophorikós* or spoken word is separated from the

[6] Richard Sherry, A *Treatise of Schemes and Tropes*, facsimile reproduction edited by Herbert W. Hildebrandt (Gainesville, 1961), p. 45.

[7] Dodd, p. 263.

lógos 'endiáthetos or meaning. Allegory as a continued metaphor requires the least shift in meaning: "from the proper signification, to another not proper, but yet nigh and like."[8] Associated with it are other forms of analogy like enigma (riddle), paroemia (proverb), and hyperbole. But the gap between the spoken word and its meaning could widen considerably; at the furthest remove one finds irony and its related forms (sarcasm and mycterismus, a more obscure form of sarcasm). In between are forms like charientismus, a kind of analogy, and diasyrmus, an ironic hyperbole. In these one person responds to another's words in a way which the speaker does not anticipate. The shift in meaning could depend upon a pun. For example, when Sir Andrew Aguecheek says that he can cut a caper, Sir Toby answers that he can cut the mutton to it (*Twelfth Night* 1. 3. 129-30). Toby has ignored the ordinary sense of the word *caper* and taken it in the sense of caper sauce. The tropological spectrum thus includes everything between analogy (allegory and enigma) and logical contraries (the ironic forms). A rough diagram of it appears on p. 60. But it is important to remember that allegory in its second sense included all these forms and could indicate anything from analogy to contradiction. This explains why Renaissance critics could reverse the meaning of an allegory when they thought it necessary, a technique which we will discuss later.

Since allegory includes the other tropes of sentences we must look briefly at them individually, for any allegorical discourse might involve them as well. We will begin with the analogical forms, using Peacham for our guide, since he has the fullest discussion of the individual tropes in English. The first of these, enigma, is simply a more obscure form of the trope, allegory. We would call it a riddle. Not many people could be expected to perceive that Peacham's example refers to fire: "As long as I liue I eate, but when I drinke I die." Fire needs matter for fuel and is extinguished by water. Peacham considers this trope more appropriate to poets than to orators, and there was certainly a

[8] Peacham, p. 3.

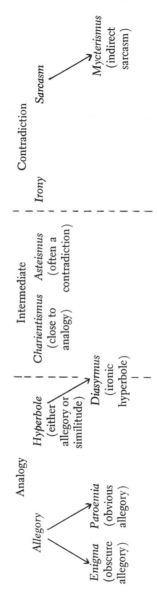

tendency among sixteenth-century poets to make their allegories
into enigmas. William Webbe confessed that he could not interpret parts of *The Shepheardes Calender,* and Chapman's
Night Poems have long been famous for their obscurity. Wilson
complains that "The misticall wisemen and Poeticall Clerkes,
will speake nothyng but quainte prouerbes, and blinde allegories,
delightyng muche in their owne darkenesse, especially, when
none can tell what thei do saie."[9] In classical times the gods used
such dark allegories in their oracular pronouncements. Apollo
advised the Athenians to flee to their wooden walls, that is, to
their fleet. Enigmatic allegory approaches most closely this oracular speech or, more precisely, the late classical idea of mythic discourse, discussed in the last chapter. It resembles divine speech
and defies human communication. Peacham quite naturally assumes that this figure agrees well with "high and heauenly
visions."

Paroemia or proverb (pár-oimos—beside the road, by the
way) is an obvious, oft-used allegory, expressed in a witty fashion.
One can formalize the relation between paroemia and enigma
by saying that when an allegory becomes too obscure it is an
enigma, and when it becomes too clear it is a proverb. Some of
Peacham's examples for this trope are still used today, but his
interpretations are quite different. He explains the famous proverb: "The tumbling stone doth seldome gather mosse" by claim-
ing that one does not gather riches and wealth by wandering.
Obviously, even in simple allegories, interpretations will vary.
Allegoric discourse is truly open-ended. What might strike us as
still more strange, Peacham considers this trope the best of all,
the most brilliant star in the tropological firmament (to use his
metaphor). He praises it so highly because it is the principal medium of moral control. He calls proverbs "The Summaries of
maners, or, The Images of humane life: for in them there is contained a generall doctrine of direction, and particular rules for all
duties in all persons." The Elizabethan dramatists' habit of end-

[9] *Arte,* f83ʳ.

ing scenes in proverbial couplets makes sense in this perspective. They were reinforcing a moral judgment to which they expected the assent of their auditors. Now, since proverb was the most potent weapon in his tropological armory, the poet had to use it sparingly and where the occasion justified it. Spenser waits until he has Red Cross trapped in the coils of a serpent before he pops in the moral: "God helpe the man so wrapt in *Errours* endlesse traine" (1. 1. 18). For modern sensibilities this proverb brings a brilliant narrative crashing down into the banal and obvious, but for Spenser the relation may have been reversed. The narrative actually justifies his moral pronouncement, which he inserts carefully into the middle of the episode as a rhetorical highlight.

Hyperbole (*úper-bállō*—to overshoot), the fourth of the analogical tropes, is not always included among them, perhaps because it often takes the form of a simile and is not, therefore, open-ended like metaphor and allegory. Peacham includes it; Sherry does not. Peacham divides up its forms in an elaborate fashion. For our purposes it suffices to say that where a comparison is made, hyperbole becomes allegory whenever one thing is equated with another, as when the lover calls his mistress an angel. When the two things are expressed by the comparative degree, a simile results. Queen Elizabeth is wiser than Pallas, or Leicester is richer than Croesus. The figure is used primarily for amplification, when the poet wishes to praise or blame a person in extreme terms. Spenser hyperbolizes his Queen as a goddess, a mirror of grace and divine majesty, and the "Great Lady of the greatest Isle" (*FQ* 1. Pro. 4). This form automatically creates explicit value judgments in the audience, as does paroemia and, in a more indirect fashion, the other tropes. One cannot speak of a person as a lion without passing a value judgment on that person. In this sense all tropological discourse functions as a medium for moral value and continues the late classical tradition, in which the poet molds the invisible standards by which his society lives. Moral exegesis is inherent in allegorical form and particularly apparent in hyperbole. Even today, Spenser's hyperbole for his

Queen: "Goddesse heauenly bright" (*FQ* 1. Pro. 4) demands the assent of an audience.

Diasyrmus (*dia-súrō*—to rip apart), a form of hyperbole sometimes included among the tropes of sentences, need not concern us here because it belongs to the low style of the satirist or the mock arguments of the Ovidian lover, as when Donne compares love to a flea. It would not appear in a serious allegory like *The Faerie Queene*.

Of the intermediate forms—charientismus and asteismus— the former relates more to analogy and the latter more to contradiction. Asteismus (*àstêlos*—urbane, clever), being confined to private discourse, is not relevant to our investigation, since all poetry is public. Charientismus (*charíeis*—graceful, elegant) mitigates hard matters with pleasant words and borders at times on flattery. The soldier who had railed against Alexander while in his cups escaped judgment by remarking that he would have said worse things, if the wine had not failed. His manner of speech softened the actual fact of his offence, while not denying it. He practiced a rough form of analogy, transposing the objectionable into the pleasant.

Of the contradictory tropes it is necessary to remember that in general no formal criteria exist for determining them. For Sherry mycterismus consists exclusively in gesture. The auditor infers the contradiction from the contrast between the speaker's statement and his facial expression. The same can apply to irony. Tropological contradiction then depends heavily upon an oral context for its effects, a good reason for modern difficulties in interpreting poetry like that of Donne, where, if it is read one way, it becomes totally serious, but read in a different tone, can only be ironic. In such a situation it is rather captious to argue whether Donne was serious or ironic, for the poem will be either once it is read. Since Renaissance theory does not recognize nonoral poetry, it follows that we can make different poems out of a single text, since we have lost the proper frame of reference to determine which version is accurate. The poem itself, as an oral product, is never both, though it may change its tone more than once during a recitation. For Peacham irony (*eirōneía*—dissimulation) is the basic form of the contradictory tropes "in which one contrarie is vnderstood by another." The auditor perceives this contradiction, as we said earlier, by observing the pronunciation of the speaker, his facial expression, or the nature of the thing referred to. Peacham's example is scriptural: "And the Lord God said, Behold, the man is become as one of vs, to know good and euill." Persistent irony must generally be avoided because it creates the impression that the speaker is a skeptic or leaves his auditors wondering when they should believe him or not. For these reasons Spenser avoids irony in *The Faerie Queene*, since he wishes to instruct his audience and wants them to trust his statements. For the same reasons the satirist habitually employs irony because he wishes to undercut his own persona.

Sarcasm (*sarkázō*—to tear flesh [*sárx*]—fressen) had the same meaning then as now, though it was reserved for more extreme circumstances, usually as a bitter taunt given to an enemy. When the Babylonians cried to the Jews "Sing vs one of your songs of Sion" they were not commending but mocking their Jewish captives. If used too often, it reflects rather on the moral condition of the speaker than on the object of his scorn. It would occur more in dramatic than poetic situations.

Mycterismus (*muktērízō*—to turn up one's nose [*muktḗr*]), the last of the tropes, can be classed as a more obscure form of sarcasm. Someone asked Demonax whether philosophers ate sweet cakes. He answered with a question: Do bees gather honey for fools only? It could take more obvious forms. Sherry suggests sticking out one's tongue.

Though allegory in its second sense could be applied to any or all of these tropes, in practice the allegorical poet confined himself to the analogical end of the spectrum. Some forms like diasyrmus and asteismus simply were not available for him to use, while the ironic forms obviated his teaching purpose. Nevertheless, the ironic forms remain important because they explain one of the stranger modes of allegorical exegesis, the notorious *lucus a non lucendo* principle. If a critic found a section of a poem which contradicted his own interpretation, he could always conclude that the section was ironic. This method would conceivably encourage wild criticism, for we would ordinarily expect an auditor to revise his interpretation before he rejected the obvious meaning of a text. But then I am not certain that the *lucus a non lucendo* principle does not operate in some literary criticism today, particularly when we wish to prove that a Renaissance poet really represented a modern outlook and saw through the illusions of his own period. In *Milton's God* (1961) Empson's reading of *Paradise Lost* provides an extended example of such ironic exegesis.

More significantly, this examination of allegory and tropology explains why the poet insisted on his moral role within society. He was not merely defending his art against its enemies, enraged at the love poems of an Ovid; he recognized the fact that morality followed inevitably from his tropological medium, morality not in the sense of current custom but in the sense of value. Every trope represents a value judgment made by comparison. No one can juxtapose a man and a toad or a man and an angel without making a moral judgment of some kind, and every trope consisted in such a juxtaposition. It could depend upon analogy or upon contradiction; in either case the medium established invisible standards. Antony's ironic moral praise, "Brutus is an honourable man,"[10] produced a moral judgment on the part of his audience just as surely as Spenser's equation of Queen Elizabeth with divine majesty. Nor could the auditor in such a situation retreat into aestheticism and avoid morality, for the poet forced his audience to cooperate with him in the very act of judgment. Spenser said Gloriana, but his audience thought of the English monarch and actually put his judgment into effect. It follows that whenever he speaks tropologically the poet must necessarily

10 *Julius Caesar* 3. 2. 92 ff.

create value, whether he wishes to or not. In allegory, then, morality is the product of language. Moral exegesis is not an optional form of interpretation; rather, it underlies the whole of allegory and, therefore, of poetry, for the two are one, as we shall see next.

In its third sense allegory was practically synonymous with poetry. More technically, it described the nature of the poet's fictions. Spenser calls *The Faerie Queene* a *continued* allegory, using the term in its precise rhetorical sense, for he wishes to distinguish his fictions from what Boccaccio calls "old wives' tales" (*GDG* 14. 9), stories which have no meaning or depth to them. Spenser's fiction is open-ended like an allegory and demands the auditor's interpretation for an adequate understanding. Spenser makes here an important distinction because the enemies of poetry did not recognize this distinction and considered all poems to be no more than literal fictions. They did not know how to analyze tropological discourse and were consequently left with contempt for poetry. They could perceive no essential difference between *The Faerie Queene* and a popular romance except for verse. Allegory then provided the poet with a precise term by which he could characterize his own fictions.

At the same time this rhetorical terminology, though undoubtedly useful, seems to dull the luster of poetry. How disappointing it is to see the mythic veil of truth dissolve into an assortment of tropological figures. But this attitude betrays our own limitations, for we have a prosaic conception of speech. The rhetorical handbooks, dreary in themselves, strengthen this attitude and make it quite difficult to see any real relationship between the poet's mystic art and a list of figures. But, here again, we tend to forget the oral context of this theory and the higher, almost ecstatic values placed upon the spoken word. The men of the Renaissance believed that the cosmos itself came into being by the spoken Word of the Lord, just as the poet creates fictional worlds through speech. By analogy one can say that the universe is God's myth and poetry man's myth. Within this context the poet's claim that his fictions are allegorical takes on fantastic proportions, for he is really arguing that his poetry has all the resonance and depth that one finds in the material cosmos. Rhetorical language allows him to be both precise and mystical about his art at one and the same time, for a trope has depth by its very definition.

The poet's use of this rhetorical terminology likewise places the entire poetic art in an oral context. No one can use such language without presupposing a speaker and an audience. The poet may not be an orator but his instinctive reliance on the technical vocabulary of the orator betrays his own attitude toward his art. For him poetry exists not in the refined, attenuated atmosphere of aesthetics but in an actual human milieu with human auditors and a social purpose. Once a living audience becomes a crucial part of the poet's consciousness, his theory must necessarily take into account practical considerations, directed toward the effects that he wishes to bring about in another human person or persons. The allegorist, for example, uses his medium to impress the images of things on the memory of his audience and at the same time forces his audience into an act of judgment. His tropological language educated his society in its traditions and reformed its morals. But we anticipate the subject of the next chapter. At the present our concern is with the implications which this oral context has for allegory or poetry considered by itself.

Even the conventional definition of poetry as allegory corresponds to an old oral definition of poetic myth. For Boccaccio, the poet "veils truth in a fair and fitting garment of fiction" (GDG 14. 7). The old definition says much the same thing: "mŷthós ĕsti lógos pseudḗs eἰkonízōn ἀlḗtheian," myth is fictional discourse imaging truth.[11] Boccaccio similarly defines in oral terms fable or fiction, by which he means allegory. He does not

[11] Roger Hinks, *Myth and Allegory in Ancient Art* (London, 1939), p. 3.

talk of it in the modern sense of the self-contained story, though
he does not deny the idea either; rather, he derives *fabula* from
a word for conversation:

> The word "fable" (*fabula*) has an honorable origin in the
> verb *for, faris*, hence "conversation" (*confabulatio*), which
> means only "talking together" (*collocutio*).
>
> [GDG 14. 9]

The word *for* itself means "to speak or say." Thus, the poet
speaks his truth orally in a tropological medium, and the auditor
fills in the unspoken parts of his analogies, re-creating within
himself the same truth.

Within their own poems the poets often exploit this familiar
atmosphere of "talking together" and address their audience
directly. In his description of the Heavenly Jerusalem, for example, Spenser apologizes to his auditors for the bareness of his
presentation because an earthly tongue cannot express it adequately (*FQ* 1. 10. 55), a conviction he reiterates in various forms
in at least ten other places.[12] Perhaps the most famous of these is
his remark which precedes the catalog of rivers and nymphs at
the wedding of the Thames and the Medway:

> All which not if an hundred tongues to tell,
> And hundred mouthes, and voice of brasse I had,
> And endlesse memorie, that mote excell,
> In order as they came, could I recount them well.
>
> [*FQ* 4. 11. 9]

In two of his Prologues he stresses the oral nature of his epic,
where he asks Queen Elizabeth to listen with a gracious ear to his
song (1. Pro. 4; 2. Pro. 5). Likewise the conventional pictures of
poets in pastorals or of the Muses generally presuppose an oral
context. It is no wonder that Stephen Hawes in the *Pastime of
Pleasure* thought a poet should learn elocution or that Ficino

---

12 *T.M.* 600; *D.* 74; *As.* 171; *FQ* 1. 11. 12; 2. 7. 19; 4. 11. 9, 44; *HL*
264; *HHB* 104, 204.

classified poetry along with music, as things apprehended by the ear.[13]

Of course, it is practically impossible to tell whether such expressions represent actual practice or just the conventional language of the poet. In two places Spenser refers specifically to reading but immediately conjoins it to speaking (*FQ* 2. 9. 60–10. 1; 3. 6. 53-54). He leaves Arthur and Guyon in the Chamber of Memory reading chronicle history but reverts to oral terminology when he describes his own poem:

> Who now shall giue vnto me words and sound,
> Equall vnto this haughtie enterprise?
>
> [*FQ* 2. 10. 1]

Did Guyon read silently or did he speak what he read? Did he read poetry or prose? These questions probably cannot be answered and are actually irrelevant because, as we have seen, poetic theory in the period depends upon an oral, not a reading, tradition. It did not recognize the fact that a man could read a poem silently. And this fact itself becomes doubtful, once we recall the well-known mellifluousness of Elizabethan verse with its lavish use of the schemes, which are purely aural figures and make no sense outside an oral context. The Elizabethan poet certainly envisaged himself as an oral artist, and he probably was so in fact.

In the instance of *The Faerie Queene* one might still argue that the allegory of the poem is much too complicated and difficult for an oral medium, however attenuated. But this objection remains theoretical and does not correspond to the actual practices of the oral poets. Some of the most difficult poetry was intended for oral performance. Riddles and guessing games form a significant portion of the oral poetry of the North, as in the Old English riddles and the verbal contentions of the *Elder Edda*. Johan Huizinga devotes a whole chapter of *Homo Ludens* to the relation between ancient poetry and this kind of play. Oral poetry

[13] See chapter 1, note 1.

seems to demand obscurity and difficulty in many of its forms: the troubadour lyric, the epic song with its kennings, the odes of a Pindar. What Spenser did was to complicate oral forms before poetic theory adjusted to the Gutenberg revolution and recognized the obsolescence of these forms. His allegory remains rooted in the oral tradition, and in its difficulties actually carries on that tradition.

Allegory, then, is an oral art in which the poet expresses a truth he has received in contemplation (GDG 14. 11) through the medium of tropological figures. The learned auditor, knowing how to interpret this kind of language, sees through the veil to the poet's own truth. He cooperates with the poet and, in a sense, completes his poem by supplying the unspoken words necessary to fill in the extended analogy of the *lógos prophorikós*. Allegory functions as the visible sign of inward truth in the poet, which the auditor expresses rationally by his interpretations. A series of equations is implied:

contemplative truth : poet
allegory : poem
multiple interpretation ("levels") : critic (auditor)

The poet must speak in allegories because the truth which he has received is inexpressible and comes to him by divine inspiration. This claim is made by most of the apologists and is not to be construed metaphorically in an age which peopled the air with *daemones* and the celestial courts with hierarchies of angels. Lodge says to Gosson that the conventional invocation of the Muse represented a real plea for the help of heaven,[14] and Boccaccio remarks that the science of poetry draws the poets "away into the region of the stars, among the divinely adorned dwellings of the gods and their heavenly splendors" (GDG 14. 4). Poetic truth is established beyond the cosmos in eternity itself.

This inspiration could be understood in two ways. Boccaccio's rhapsodic descriptions apply rather to biblical literature,

14 In Smith, 1: 72.

which he considers to be a form of poetry. The Greek poets had no divine inspiration; they participated in it indirectly by imitating the Hebrews, and were directly "prompted by mere energy of mind" (GDG 14. 8). Poetry as a whole might stream forth "from the bosom of God" (GDG 14. 7), but the individual poet might be gifted only in a natural way according to the old commonplace: "Poeta nascitur, orator fit." Genius guarantees ability to the poet, but not truth, for which he needs literary imitation. Golding maintains a similar position and argues at length in his Epistle to Leicester that Ovid imitated Genesis in his accounts of Creation and the Flood (332-540). The Florentines were more extreme in their contentions: Homer had a divine revelation as well as Moses, only of a lesser degree. In this perspective the poet becomes another Hermes, guiding the souls of men into another world, and the clear springs of Helicon redden with the blood of the Titans.[15] All the old conventions of priestly rhetoric revive, and the auditor can hope again to scale Olympus through poetry. Revelation awaits the few who ponder over the poet's sayings.

Ficino, in a letter to Alexander Braccius, appeals to the *Ion* for his evidence that the poet is inspired by God.[16] The divine spirit manifests its presence visibly as a *furor* or rapture, transferred by the poet to his auditors by means of his spoken words. Politian gives an elaborate description of this *furor* in the *Nutricia* (182 ff). The poets themselves wonder at the oracles they have expressed while possessed by the spirit. Their minds become darkened to visible objects, and they cannot stop themselves from speaking. After the fit a quiet follows and their mouths become silent. But the songs they have committed to fragile papyrus will blow the same Apolline raptures thousands of years later and will breathe on the musical strings of heaven. During such a recitation a holy contagion will possess the audience, the *furor* from the poet's breast burning itself into them, and they will all be-

---

15 Reynolds quotes Pico to this effect. See Spingarn, 1: 151.
16 *Opera omnia* 1. 2. 673.

come united within the poet's spirit, like a magnet which holds together a whole chain of iron links. In one of his prologues to *The Faerie Queene* Spenser uses this technical language. The Muses have infused into his mind a "goodly fury" and guide him into strange ways. No one can find these paths by himself, for the Muses must lead him.

Allegory, then, depends upon inspiration or *furor*, and this conception of inspiration likewise provides a rationale for the polysemous or allegorical readings of a critic. Both the poet and his auditor have difficulty in explaining tropological discourse, once the *furor* is passed. They may have apprehended the same truth, but they will explain it differently. The various levels of allegory represent the attempts by critics to represent this truth in rational terms. They cannot rest content with a single explanation because the allegorical truth, which they wish to define, is inexpressible and is experienced in rapture rather than by reason. Modern analogies might help us understand this process somewhat better. For Eliot the poem should stimulate in the reader an objective correlative of the poet's original sensation, an essentially drier description of the same poetic action, with the ecstatic elements removed. And Eliot tried to encourage a polysemous interpretation of his poems by refusing to explain them. Rilke waxes more eloquent. In a letter to Princess Marie he characterizes the completion of the *Duino Elegies* in terms of *furor:*[17]

> All in a few days, there was a nameless storm, a hurricane, in my mind (like that time in Duino), everything in the way of fibre and web in me split,—eating was not to be thought of, God knows who fed me.
> But now IT IS. IS.
> Amen.

Such analogies indicate that the Renaissance notion of inspiration in allegory is by no means confined to its period, but they can also be misleading because they ignore the oral nature of the

[17] *Duino Elegies*, ed. and trans. J. B. Leishman and Stephen Spender (New York, 1939), p. 13.

poetic action in the sixteenth century, and it is this oral context, once more, which requires an alteration of perspective on our part when we approach an allegory like *The Faerie Queene*.

First of all, we cannot expect from Renaissance allegory the close-knit unity one associates with Aristotelian drama or some kinds of poetry. Ariosto's episodic tale was recited in parts, the whole being much too long for a single recitation. The same applies to *The Faerie Queene*. Spenser could anticipate a segmented understanding of his complex epic and did not have to tidy up his story. His audience would remember certain episodes and certain characters, and they would respond to the reiteration of certain themes, but they could never be expected to recall the details of his plot. They would inevitably confuse characters and episodes. For example, one student I knew, who was reading Malory, could remember the adventure on the ship in the Grail narrative and could distinguish sharply a Lancelot from a Galahad, but he could not recall who entered the ship. The most an allegorical poet could do was to impose a loose kind of thematic unity on his story, of the sort that William Nelson examines throughout his *Poetry of Edmund Spenser* (1963). Even if he constructed a careful plot, his industry would have no particular value in his rhetorical situation. What he could anticipate in his audience was a general understanding of the main narrative thread and an intense concentration on individual episodes, and this is precisely what Renaissance commentaries reveal: either an elaborate discussion of individual events or an overall concern for the total myth.

Second, we must alter slightly our ideas of textual commentaries. They were not exclusively an exegesis; they also provided the auditor with the necessary lore to appreciate a poem while it was recited. Renaissance poets were only too conscious of the difficulties created by their tropological medium, and they resorted to extratextual means to keep open the communication with their audience. The commentaries performed this role. In the case of a new poem, the poet often took care that a letter or commentary of some sort was added to it, "knowing how doubt-fully all Allegories may be construed" (Letter to Raleigh). Spen-ser had E. K. interpret his *Shepheardes Calender* and prefaced *The Faerie Queene* with his own explanatory letter. Boccaccio likewise disclosed the secrets of his *Eclogues* in a letter to Fra Martino da Signa.[18] Such interpretations did not replace the poem, for the poet usually left many guidelines for his hearers in the form of proverbs and explicit statements. Rather, they indi-cated the learning necessary to any person who wished to under-stand the poem properly. They were propaedeutic as well as exegetical.

In conclusion, one might say that the term *allegory*, in what-ever sense it is used, invariably presupposes an oral situation. In poetry the allegorical figures make up the garment of truth, which the auditor unravels—almost futilely because he will never find an ultimate interpretation. The poet's truth defies rational ex-pression; no number of interpretations will suffice. But this total act of creation and analysis must have a purpose; and, since it exists in an oral context, this purpose must be practical. It must involve human beings in a significant fashion and for an im-portant end. Allegory is intimately associated with the society in which the poet writes; it demands human participation and must be explicable in social terms. Here again, the oral context of al-legorical theory becomes necessary, for the purposes of this tropological rhetoric are largely memorial, a factor which remains inexplicable for people brought up with large libraries and thou-sands of printed books. A poet like Edmund Spenser really tried to play the role of a Homer for his own society, an attempt in which he failed. Why he failed and what he made of his failure belong to the next chapter, where we will discuss the memorial purpose of allegorical rhetoric.

[18] In the *Opere Latine Minori*, ed. A. F. Massèra (Bari, 1928), p. 216.

4

The Purpose of Allegory: Its Memorial Role in Society

Their whole . . . life is a commemoration, a remembering.   Mircea Eliade[1]

WITHIN SOCIETY the poet had for his purpose the moral education of his contemporaries, which he effected in a Homeric manner by impressing upon their memories lively images of the various forms of moral conduct. Spenser wanted to portray in his *Faerie Queene* the private virtues of a gentleman and had in mind yet another epic devoted to public virtues. Like Homer he tried to create a kind of moral encyclopedia for his society, and like Homer he envisaged his auditors carrying around this encyclopedia within the memory chambers of their own minds. The Renaissance poet identified memory training with education and still used Hesiod's old oral myth, which told how poetry grew out of memory.[2] For him the purposes of poetry remained Homeric, despite all the manifest differences that we might observe between the rhetorical situation of Spenser and that of Homer. Hesiod's myth was already more than two thousand years old and the conditions of society had radically changed. In the Renaissance the educated individual did not have to remember all he knew, for he could always check his books or manuscripts for whatever information he required. Some people even amassed

[1] *The Sacred and the Profane*, trans. Willard R. Trask (New York, 1961), p. 101.
[2] See in particular the early chapters in Eric Havelock's *Preface to Plato* (Cambridge, Mass., 1963).

relatively large libraries. The allegorical poet, though unconscious of the significance of this technological change, nevertheless realized with some intensity that the times had changed, and he had already developed a different explanation for his memorial role in society, drawing upon psychological theory, highly developed memory techniques, and Platonism, all of which had developed since the age of oral poetry as we understand the term. It will be our purpose to show first how the allegorical poets understood in psychological terms Hesiod's oral myth, which told how poetry grew out of memory. Afterward, we can discuss the careful devices of imagery used by the Renaissance poet to affect the human memory, the moral and educational purposes which these devices served, and the memorial-historical framework in which they were put. We will begin with Hesiod's myth.

As Hesiod tells the story, Zeus slept nine nights with Mnemosyne in her bed remote from the immortals; and a year later she bore him nine daughters, the Muses, who went to their father on snowy Olympus:[3]

> and the dark earth resounded about them as they chanted and a lovely sound rose up beneath their feet as they went to their father. And he was reigning in heaven, himself holding the lightning and glowing thunderbolt, when he had overcome by might his father Cronos. . . .

Hesiod, by assigning the Muses to Zeus, the judge and ruler of a newly conquered universe, indicated the governing and formative role poetry had for his society, and by Mnemosyne the essential part memory had in it. Roger Hinks explains this conception in modern terms:[4]

> . . . without memory, civilized life is impossible, for memory is the prerequisite condition for that mental coherence which distinguishes human consciousness in the higher sense from the mere animal awareness of the brute creation. It is the

---

[3] *Theogeny* 69-73.
[4] *Myth and Allegory*, p. 93.

possession of a memory that makes man a historical being; and it is the faculty for being historical that gives him a personality.

The oral poet: "chants the glorious deeds of men of old and the blessed gods who inhabit Olympus. . . ." (*Theogeny* 100-101). He recalls the past, acting as memory for society.

Renaissance mythographers interpreted this fable psychologically. For Natalis Comes, memory strengthens the knowledge which the poet receives from God. Boccaccio has a more precise explanation. Memory makes communication itself possible. The poet, though he may have divine knowledge, depends on his memory to share it with others; for without memory, his vision remains shut up within himself and can have no value for others. In Persius' phrase: "Scire tuum nil est, nisi scire hoc te sciat alter." It is not enough to know something; another must know that you know it.[5] In other words, whatever visions or insights the poet might have, they will remain socially useless and will not justify his poetry unless he stores them carefully in his memory so that on a later occasion he can retell them to others. A rather rudimentary and obvious idea, but it has extensive implications. Spenser's Arthur and Guyon find their national histories written in the memory of the human soul, as Spenser himself finds the stories of *The Faerie Queene* in his Muse's document chest—that is, in his own mind.[6] The memory on which poetic communication depends must be little less than extraordinary.

For the poet, memory was the necessary precondition of his delivery; for his audience, its result. An allegorical critic like Sir John Harington saw in poetry a kind of moral and social mnemonics:[7]

> another cause why they wrote in verse was conseuration of the memorie of their precepts, as we see yet the generall rules

[5] Giovanni Boccaccio *Genealogie deorum gentilium* 11. 2. Natalis Comes *Mythologiae* 7. 15.

[6] For Spenser, see *FQ* 1. Pro. 2; 2. 9-10.

[7] From his Preface to the *Orlando Furioso*, p. 203 Smith, vol. 2.

almost of euerie art, not so much as husbandrie, but they are oftner recited and better remembred in verse then in prose.

Today we still use the old memory jingle: "Thirty days hath September,/April, June, and November." Hence, perhaps, the plethora of "sentences" and aphorisms in Renaissance poetry. These short, often obvious, statements were intended to be memorized by the reader. Ficino argues in one of his letters that song can aid memory by the delight and admiration it causes. Delight incites genius, feeds the will and strengthens the memory itself; through admiration the mind becomes more deeply attentive and burns the marks of things on its own inner chambers.[8]

Allegory itself duplicated these metrical effects and strengthened one's memory. Peacham remarks that the efficient cause of a metaphor and, therefore, of an allegory is the judgment and memory of the writer; and among its final causes or purposes, he lists the pleasure it gives to the reader's judgment and the lively images of things it imprints on his memory.[9] Metaphoric speech requires in both poet and audience a combination of memory and judgment, of Zeus and Mnemosyne. Unlike the philosopher, who appeals only to Zeus and carefully excludes Mnemosyne from his imageless discourse, the poet needs the goddess for the very definition of his art, where thought and image are united.

The specific techniques by which the poet affected the memories of his audience were themselves invented by a poet; for the art of memory, as begun by Simonides and elaborated by the classical rhetoricians, merely consisted in a kind of unspoken allegory. Since Frances Yates has already examined this technique of putting images into mental places, I will cover the matter only briefly. Thomas Wilson's orator uses an allegorical bedroom scene to keep in mind an incredible lawsuit brought against a client, who was accused simultaneously of theft, adultery, riot, manslaughter, and treason. In various parts of the room

---

[8] *Opera omnia* 1. 2. 656.
[9] Peacham, *Garden*, pp. 3-4, 13-14.

he puts notable examples of each crime, like Venus for adultery
and Richard III for manslaughter.[10] Magicians like Giordano
Bruno were more ambitious; they replaced the bedroom with the
cosmos and put archetypal images on concentric wheels, by virtue
of which the mind of the magus both reflected and controlled
the universe.[11] With either Wilson or Bruno the art of memory
consists in a kind of allegory, because the person learns to find
ideas in concrete images, much as a critic might interpret a set
scene in Spenser, like the pageant of the seasons and the months.
Since Renaissance critics habitually identified allegory with
poetry, a series of equivalences is suggested: memory with allegory and both with poetry.

In their own writings the allegorical poets constantly practiced Simonides' memory techniques. Frances Yates argues that
Dante made the whole *Divine Comedy* into a series of such
mnemonic images inserted into mental places,[12] and Spenser
and Hawes provide some Renaissance examples. In the *Pastime
of Pleasure* Graunde Amoure encounters the Seven Liberal Arts
in seven successive chambers of the Tower of Doctrine. That of
Rhetoric is strewn with flowers, the perfumes of which:

> . . . dyde well encense out
> All mysty vapours/ of perturbacyon.
>
> [661-62]

Mirrors cover the walls, and the lady herself sits in a high chair,
wearing a "vesture/ clerely puryfyed" (656), with the emblematic
laurel garland over her head. Here Hawes has created a memory
room by which his readers can recall the essential qualities of
rhetoric: invention and style, the mirrors and the flowers.
Spenser has many such rooms and images in *The Faerie Queene*,
employing the *imagines agentes* recommended in the *Rhetorica
ad Herennium*, which depend upon a complex application of

[10] Wilson, f109^v-110^r.

[11] See Frances Yates' discussion of *De umbris idearum* in *The Art of
Memory* (Chicago, 1966), pp. 199-230.

[12] Ibid., pp. 95-96.

memory techniques and, therefore, require some explanation. The mind itself seldom remembers ordinary occurrences; it needs the novel and the unusual to create enough of an impression so that it will never forget the event. The extraordinary happening, whether ridiculous, dishonorable, great, or unbelievable, remains impressed on the memory. One recalls incidents from childhood so clearly because they were experienced before the individual had become habituated to certain kinds of phenomena, which later will pass by unnoticed. A sunrise or sunset, no matter how beautiful, fails to impress a mature mind, since it happens every day, while a solar eclipse creates wonder, more so even than an eclipse of the moon, which one sees more often. Thus, in the experience of natural events, the artist finds the basis for an effective memory technique. He imitates nature, looking for strange and unusual images, the kind which will remain longest in the memory. For this purpose he uses a few striking images; few because too many will dull the mind, made to expect and therefore to ignore even unusual images, when they are everywhere present. These images must likewise be vivid and dramatic, for who can remember the vague? As a result, the artist must make images of extreme beauty or ugliness, and each of them must be ornamented with a distinguishing trait: a crown or purple cloak, something comic or ridiculous, or something very ugly. He can disfigure an image, painting it in glaring colors, covering it with mud, or staining it with blood. Reality and art must obey the same principle: the unusual is the stimulus of the powers of memory.[13]

For Spenser's application of this particular memory technique one need only recall Amoret stumbling along in Cupid's pageant, with her breast ripped open and her heart laid in a silver basin, transfixed by a dart. Or there is Spenser's own picture of Memory. He makes Memory an infinitely old man, decrepit in body though lively in mind, sitting in a chamber which mirrors his state; for, while it appears "ruinous and old," it has

---

[13] Ibid., pp. 9-10, paraphrased from the Hubbell translation in the Loeb edition.

firm, strong walls. Old books and long parchment scrolls, worm-eaten and full of canker holes, cover the walls. Memory sits in a chair, tossing and turning his documents, helped by a little boy called Anamnestes, who fetches whatever the old man wants and looks around for anything which may have been lost or mislaid among all the books and manuscripts.[14] Now it would be very difficult to forget such a graphic picture. This terribly old man, fumbling among his worm-eaten manuscripts, will remain in one's memory long after the specific episode of Guyon and Arthur in Book II may either have been forgotten or have become confused with other tales in *The Faerie Queene*. At the same time Spenser's picture of Memory, as we shall see later, contains a considerable amount of information about the mnemonic process and is crucial for our understanding of Renaissance theory.

When the allegorical poet stimulated and controlled the memories of his audience, he was emulating the moral and educational role which the oral poet held in ancient society. His memory images had a moral, doctrinal purpose; they civilized his audience. Orpheus had brought a "rude and sauage people to a more ciuill and orderly life," and the allegorical poet had the same function:[15]

> Carbuncles/in the most derke nyght
> Doth shyne fayre/with clere radyant beames
> Exylynge derkenes/with his rayes lyght
> And so these poetes/with theyr golden streames
> Deuoyde our rudenes/with grete fyry lemes.

The precise content of this moral education is rather the subject of the next chapter, where the moral level of allegory will be discussed. Here our principal concern is with the mode in which poets communicated this morality.

They usually set their moral instructions within a mnemonic-historical framework. The oral poet "chants the glorious deeds

---

[14] *FQ* 2. 9. 55-58.
[15] Puttenham, *Arte* 1. 3, p. 6; and Hawes, 1128-32.

of men of old and the blessed gods who inhabit Olympus . . ."
(*Theogeny* 100-101), selecting out of the past appropriate material with which he creates standards in the present. In the
same manner Spenser sings of "Knights and Ladies gentle deeds"
(*FQ* 1. Pro. 1), which he pretends have remained forgotten for
a millenium. In his own picture of Memory, which we have
already discussed, Spenser explains this technique. The old man
remembers the whole of human history: the Trojan War, the
wars of King Ninus, even the dim past before the Deluge, for
he recalls the infancy of Methuselah. For Spenser the human
memory is essentially communal and general, including everything significant which man has done since the beginning of
time. Accordingly, the poet can assume that his audience will be
able to recall the same public events he does; they both remember the common human past.

The poet likewise places the present under the rule of memory, as Pindar explains:[16]

> Even high deeds of prowess
> Have a great darkness if they lack song,
> We can hold up a mirror to fine doings
> In one way only,
> If with the help of Memory in her glittering crown
> Recompense is found for labour
> In words' echoing melodies.

Bowra's note deserves quotation: "Song is a mirror not only
because it reflects but because it keeps the essential brightness of
noble achievements." The present aspires to the condition of a
glorious past, and the poet selects out of the present what corresponds to his ancient standards. Consequently, Mnemosyne
immortalizes the present in terms of the past. Pindar turns his
athletic victors into the heroes of old; and Spenser transforms
Queen Elizabeth into "That greatest Glorious Queene" of Arthurian days (1. 1. 3), asking her to see in this past a mirror of
the present (2. Pro. 4):

[16] Quoted by C. M. Bowra in *Pindar* (Oxford, 1964), p. 10.

And thou, O fairest Princesse vnder sky,
In this faire mirrhour maist behold thy face,
And thine owne realmes in lond of Faery,
And in this antique Image thy great auncestry.

Spenser can use King Arthur as a standard for his own day, because he realizes that through memory the past continues to have a kind of existence in the present; the ancient heroes live on in the minds of those who remember them. We have already noted that in his picture of Memory Spenser has the old man recall everything significant which ever happened. Within his own consciousness the old man gives to the past an eternal presentness or immortality. Whatever was, is in the memory.

Even the future comes under Memory's rule. The Muses breathed into Hesiod "a divine voice to celebrate things that shall be and things that were aforetime" (*Theogeny* 31-32). The paradoxical claim that the poet knows the future by *recalling* it at least tries to explain actual facts. Daniel *saw* a vision of the four beasts which were to come,[17] and John saw the world die on Patmos. Spenser may be hinting at the Renaissance interpretation of this paradox when he makes the old man in his picture half-blind. Blindness was a traditional sign of inner vision. The Muse who helped Homer's Demodokos to perceive the good and evil of life and made him into a poet had at the same time deprived him of his sight. Renaissance critics believed that Homer himself had paid the same price for his interior vision, as did the prophet Tiresias, who saw Pallas or Ideal Beauty naked and consequently became blind to the sensible world. By his experience he gained a knowledge of all things, past and future.[18] Through

---

[17] Daniel 7.
[18] *Odyssey* 8. 62-64, in Fitzgerald's translation (New York, 1961):

> The crier soon came, leading that man of song
> whom the Muse cherished; by her gift he knew
> the good of life, and evil—
> for she who lent him sweetness made him blind.

For Homer and Tiresias see Henry Reynolds' paraphrase of Pico della Mirandola in Spingarn, 1: 151.

the same mode of vision he knew everything. This notion invites a Platonic interpretation, which we will discuss later. At present, it suffices to say that through memory the poet breaks out of the world of time into a kind of extratemporal viewpoint, from which past and future are seen to form different parts of a common human pattern.

Allegory and poetry civilize men because the present is judged implicitly or explicitly in relation to a mythic past, which itself possesses a transcendent perfection and can apply to any stage of human history. The art of poetry "offers to wretched mortals higher things than the mind can grasp, better things than impiety can desire, greater things than human weakness dares to accomplish."[19] Moral criticism follows necessarily from poetry's basis in memory and judgment; or, in other words, Mnemosyne makes possible judgment in the poet's audience, and hence, social improvement. The contrast between the glorious past and the mundane present stirs men up to judge themselves and try to recapture the ancient virtues. The poets were "the first priests, the first prophets, the first Legislators and polititians in the world," as well as the "first Philosophers, the first Astronomers and Historiographers and Oratours and Musitiens."[20]

It is clear then that the allegorical poet of the Renaissance, filled with the belief that he was practicing the same oral art his predecessors had used two thousand years before, wanted to emulate the role of a Homer. More frequently, of course, he talked of Virgil, whom he understood in the same fashion, though a modern would distinguish the two. Virgil was already removed from the purely oral conditions of Homeric society, but the Renaissance poet ascribed to both artists the responsibilities of an oral educator. The Renaissance poet tried to do everything for his own society that Homer had done for eighth-century Greece, a task which was primarily understood in terms of education. Through memory the poet governed society, exercising a

[19] John Rainolds, *Oratio*, p. 39.
[20] From the titles for Puttenham, 1. 3-4.

kind of cultural control over men's minds. For this end he had created a highly developed image technique based on a psychology of memory and designed to establish the standards by which men judged things. This psychology was communal and general; the poet appealed not to the peculiar psychological traits of the individual but to those traits common to all men. Thus he drew upon history, the record of public events, for his material, exploiting the memory of humanity itself and selecting out of the mass of historical events those which he judged appropriate for his educational purposes. *The Faerie Queene* as much as the *Iliad* was designed to civilize and educate human society.

II

All this imitation by the allegorical writer of oral poetry cannot mask a crucial difference between the two. In blunt terms the oral poet succeeded in his endeavors and the allegorical poet failed. In fact, the more the allegorist relied upon memory, the more isolated he found himself to be in society, for the values he revived from the past did not correspond to contemporary norms. Worse, there was a group of pseudopoets who wrote verse and who, like the orators, exploited the commonplaces of their own day, ignoring memory altogether. Henry Reynolds in *Mythomystes* called them "pretenders to Poesy" and compared their creations to Ixion's cloud.[21] Writers like George Gascoigne in his *Adventures of F. J.* were displacing the older poets and usurping their role. Now the allegorical poet had to explain his failure in some fashion. A modern might explain his lack of success by saying that he was using outmoded principles for his art, principles designed for oral conditions either in the process of rapid decay or already dead. The alphabet had long ago made oral poetry obsolescent, and whatever oral characteristics may have survived the change could not stand against the printed

[21] In Spingarn, 1: 148. Ixion tried to seduce Juno but instead made love to a cloudy counterfeit.

book. A person with a large library does not need an oral poet to develop his memory. But the Renaissance poets could not be expected to understand their failure in such terms; they had to think in the modes of their own day and they found answers for their problem in a moral analysis of society and in the Platonism which was popular in the period. The former demonstrated why society as a whole rejected them; the latter, why a few did listen. The poets were forced eventually to conclude that they did in fact, like Homer, appeal to humanity but that most people chose to ignore their peculiarly human traits and therefore had no time for the allegorical poet.

The Renaissance poet perceived in his audience a moral condition which separated it essentially from the audience of the old oral poet. The people in the audience of the oral poet were either just acquiring the values and practices of civilization or were strengthening them in their memories, while the allegorical poet had to contend with people who had already forgotten these values and had no desire to recall them. In Politian's explanation God originally sent poetry down to primeval man, uncivilized, without ritual, knowledge, or social organization. Poetry or "this heavenly animal," as Politian calls it, awakened in early man his weak mind and heart, feeble from a long sleep, and became the mistress and charioteer of his soul.[22] But in the Renaissance, man no longer wished to hear the voice of poetry and manufactured pseudopoets, versifiers without divine inspiration or a sense for true values, to praise the status quo—that is, to justify his own lapsed state. Spenser has Calliope lament that her patrons no longer care to have the ancestry of the old heroes memorialized anew nor do they want others to remember them. They prefer to have the heroes forgotten, as they themselves will be forgotten. In effect, they want man to live completely without memory, the medium of moral value. Peacham in the *Compleat Gentleman* asks himself a related question: why are poets no

[22] *Nutricia*, 34-115, in *Le Selve e La Strega*, ed. Isidoro del Lungo (Florence, 1925).

longer esteemed? He answers that virtue receives no regard in a declining and corrupt society, and he quotes Pietro Aretino, who remarks wryly that princes do not patronize poets because they realize how unworthy they are of the praises given them by poets.[23] What is still more serious, people have actually turned the moral world upside down. In his Prologue to the Fifth Book of *The Faerie Queene* Spenser argues that what used to be called virtue is now called vice and what was formerly vice is now termed virtue. Right is now wrong and wrong has become right. Everything has been totally reversed.

The corruption of society is a great commonplace in allegorical criticism; Hawes, Nashe, Spenser, and Reynolds all dwell upon it.[24] Ignorance has caused this decay; the poet must reawaken his contemporaries to ancient values, and, therefore, is forced backward into history for appropriate material, as Spenser explains:

> Let none then blame me, if in discipline
>   Of vertue and of ciuill vses lore,
>   I doe not forme them to the common line
>   Of present dayes, which are corrupted sore,
>   But to the antique vse, which was of yore,
>   When good was onely for it selfe desyred.
>   [FQ 5, Pro. 3]

The poet tries to evoke communal memories of a virtuous past.

Before he could recall the ancient attitudes to the minds of his audience, he had to memorize them himself by assiduous study of the older poets. Hawes professed himself a disciple of Lydgate; and E. K. in his Preface to *The Shepeardes Calender* made Spenser a student of Chaucer and his contemporaries, whom he read so thoroughly that he picked up their phrases and language almost by accident, making them a part of his own spirit. His

[23] Spenser, *Teares*, 439-44; Peacham, *The Compleat Gentleman*, in Spingarn, 1: 120.

[24] *Pastime*, 1275-88. For Nashe see the selection in Smith, 1; for Reynolds, in Spingarn, 1: 144-45.

celebrated archaic style indicated what he had become through his reading, like a man walking in the sun who gets sunburned. His style manifested not so much deliberate and conscious experiment as his own individual spirit, molded in the antique tradition. Unfortunately, this practice of imitation further isolated the poet from the society he was trying to educate. From his study of older poetry Spenser had learned values quite alien to his contemporaries, and these values manifested themselves in a style still more alien to normal modes of speech. He could hardly expect an enthusiastic response from his audience, when both his style and his point of view differed so radically from the ordinary. The more he attempted to carry on the traditional functions of poetry, the more barriers he set up which blocked his way to the achievement of those ends.

The pseudopoets knew better. They used the older poets rather as a quarry for useful phrases and topics, in the same way as a rhetorician might use a handbook of commonplaces and well-known aphorisms. They never tried to recover the spirit of the older poetry and never lost themselves in outmoded speech forms. For the allegorist such practices violated the whole purpose of imitation, because they did not enlarge one's memory. Reynolds complains that even the rack would never get the pseudopoets to confess to more than a superficial imitation. They copied the style and phrases of an older author but did not recall his point of view.[25] Such imitation had grave consequences for the kind of poetry they wrote, which itself became superficial. The pseudopoets had to depend upon their own minds for the substance of their poetry, since they were unwilling to understand the older poets; and the individual mind is limited where the mind of humanity is not. Through memory the individual poet establishes communication with the greatness of spirit which informs the writings of earlier artists and thinkers; and he can, therefore, broaden and heighten the powers of his own mind and develop some sensible standards of conduct.

[25] Spingarn, 1: 148.

And yet the pseudopoets could defend their misuse of literary imitation, for they could at least reach a wider audience, though they might have nothing to say to them. For the allegorist the situation was an impossible one. If he wanted to write significant poetry, he had to immerse himself in his own memory of the older tradition; but the more he did so, the smaller his audience became.

In fact, the allegorical poet found himself in much the same position as the old prophets. Faced with a diminutive audience, he went on uttering truths quite alien to his contemporaries and ended up causing a moral change only within a few. The more he tried, the less success he had. Unlike the allegorists of antiquity he did not really speak to two audiences, providing moral control for the many and instruction for the few; even his moral message was restricted to the few. The ordinary critic of Tudor England understood this situation (though he may not have thought about the prophetic analogy), and he customarily identified the moral level of allegory with its inner meaning, an identification which a Julian would never have made, nor for that matter a Pico della Mirandola, who sharply distinguished the moral function of allegory from its profounder message. Spenser, who had both depth and morality in his poetry, nevertheless explained his *Faerie Queene* in strictly moral terms, following the conventional line and giving implicit recognition to his rhetorical dilemma, which he evaluated explicitly in the Prologue to Book Five. The Renaissance poet found himself in the old prophetic cul-de-sac and could find no way out of it.

In this unhappy situation the allegorical poet looked back with nostalgia and envy to the days when an Orpheus or an Amphion had received such general recognition in society. The stones and trees listened to Orpheus, but the allegorists could not move the stony men of their own time.[26] Instead they constantly had to defend poetry against the attacks of critics, who hated the abuses of the pseudopoets and refused to distinguish

[26] The phrase is Spenser's in *FQ* 5. Pro. 2.

them from the true. Indifference was a still greater enemy; few cared enough about poetry to patronize it. In a society of virtuous vices, false art, and general disinterest, how could the poet expect to make his voice heard, and who would listen? Spenser himself suggests an answer in a passage from his Platonic *Hymne to Love*, where he clarifies the relation of judgment to memory, the two powers which, as we have seen, make poetry possible. He is trying to explain why the lover responds to beauty and says:

> For hauing yet in his deducted spright,
> Some sparks remaining of that heauenly fyre,
> He is enlumind with that goodly light,
> Vnto like goodly semblant to aspyre:
> Therefore in choice of loue, he doth desyre
> That seemes on earth most heauenly, to embrace,
> That same is Beautie, borne of heauenly race.
>
> [106-12]

Memory makes judgment possible; the lover chooses what he finds corresponds to the sparks of heavenly fire which enlighten his own mind. For the poet this principle means that he can expect a response only from those who are like him, from those who are willing to share in his vision because they judge things by the same standards, and these standards exist in the memory. The individual judges objects by the sparks of fire which still remain in him; he recalls true beauty and therefore can recognize it when he sees it.

This theory of judgment presupposes the Platonic doctrine of anamnesis, a quite natural connection for the allegorical poet to make; for a poetic which places so much emphasis on memory would necessarily express itself philosophically in a system which similarly stresses memory and provides a rationale for it. Allegorical theory practically demands Platonism for its understanding, or rather Neoplatonism, since the Renaissance Platonists read their master by means of Plotinus and Proclus. With the help of Platonism the poet can equate his Mnemosyne with the anamnesis of the philosophers and therefore can understand his role in society more precisely and can reconcile himself to his apparent failure; for his own purposes necessitate it. He does not in fact control the morals of his society; rather, he is trying to reform them.

The identification of Mnemosyne with anamnesis might at first glance seem to create certain difficulties, because Mnemosyne concerns herself essentially with historical events, while in anamnesis the individual recalls a prehistorical situation, something which he knew before he entered the world of time and history. But, as we have seen, the poet does much the same thing when, by recalling both the past and the future, he participates in a viewpoint somehow beyond time, concerned though it may be with events in time or expressing itself through them. The Platonic anamnesis can function in like fashion, for in the *Symposium* Plato finds mythic truth through history. The dialogue is a gigantic exercise in oral recall. Apollodorus begins it by telling a companion of his about a feast at Agathon's which occurred a long time ago. He himself had not been there, but he had heard about it from Aristodemus who had, and he had checked certain parts of Aristodemus' story with Socrates. Now Apollodorus cannot remember everything which Aristodemus said, nor could Aristodemus remember everything which happened at the banquet, but Apollodorus will recall whatever he considers worthy of remembrance (*Symposium* 178). As with the poet, Memory selects for Apollodorus only the significant aspects of past events, not the trivial. In the middle of the feast this memorial act recurs, throwing the history still further into the past and giving it a mythic character. Socrates tells his drinking companions a tale that he learned many years before from the wise woman, Diotima of Mantineia. This myth about the birth of Eros reveals an unchanging truth and provides the basis for a dialectic by which the individual can recover truth beyond time. Truth then appears in history at the point where a modern historian would find the mythic and the legendary, because it de-

pends upon hearsay and cannot be verified. Plato recounts
for his readers the words of Apollodorus, who recalls the
words of Aristodemus, who repeats as best he can the words of
Socrates, who in turn is recalling the words of Diotima. Similarly, Homer recalls the fabulous exploits of the heroes at Troy
and Spenser the legendary achievements of King Arthur, both
of which occurred in the remote past and yet reveal a kind of
mythic truth. Both the poet's Mnemosyne and the philosopher's
anamnesis presuppose the coexistence of transtemporal truth
and historical event. The philosopher departs from the ways of
the poet when he tries to abstract truth from event and creates
a discourse without images and not dependent upon memory.
He may learn through memory but rejects her power in his own
mode of expression.

The Orphic *Hymn to Mnemosyne* well expresses the specific
function of Platonic memory within the communication established between the poet and his audience. Invoked as the goddess who joins the soul to a higher intelligence, Mnemosyne
breaks the chains of Lethe and awakens the mental eye from its
long sleep in oblivion's darkness.[27] Thus, one can say that memory turns the eye of the soul back to the light of Spenser's
heavenly fire, or in broader terms, allegory wakens the soul from
the dream of life.[28] The poet stirs the memories of his audience
to recall their true nature and their lost home, and he can evoke
this reminiscence because he has already experienced it himself;
that is, memory is still both an efficient and a final cause of his
art. The poet heard through the cracks and fissures of his bodily
prison images of the celestial music he had known long ago,
before his mind descended into matter; and, wishing to see the
old vision again, he tried to fly back home but found he could

[27] Adapted from the translation by Thomas Taylor in his *Hymns of
Orpheus* (London, 1792).
[28] The first phrase is from Taylor's commentary to the *Hymn*, p. 76;
the second, from André Chastel's *Marsile Ficin et L'Art* (Geneva, 1954),
p. 147.

not. Failing to actualize the past, he imitated the music of his vision, to communicate it to others, and created a discourse made up of images designed to engrave the delphic senses of the mind.[29] Allegorical poetry, then, memorializes the poet's vision, while it signifies the poet's failure to escape from matter. What the poet awakes in his audience is the same vision he and everyone else once had. Again the memorial act is communal.

The pseudopoet weaves his allegorical web out of his own mind, for he has not recalled the ancient vision. He thus produces empty poetry, without depth; he stirs no one's memories. Or in the language of the oral poet, the Muses can tell "false things as though they were true" as well as true things (*Theogeny* 27). True poetry combines *sophía* and *téchnē*, wisdom and art; false poetry has only *téchnē*, images without vision, art without inspiration.[30] It is not the child of Mnemosyne.

It is within this context of Platonic thought that the poet can finally understand his own failure with some precision. He can recognize the fact that few people have even the capacity to recall his vision; they pursue external beauty and ignore the mind. As a result, the allegorical poet can never have a large audience. Most have allowed the sparks of heavenly fire within them to die out and have nothing for the poet to rekindle. Therefore, they can never break through the poet's allegory to the vision which occasioned it. They are aliens and strangers to the poet, people who cannot recognize his standards or values, since they have never used memory to explore the depths of their own personalities and consequently regard everything else superficially. For them the poet's allegory remains a painted veil, impenetrable to their eyes, for they have never learned to look at things properly. They exist without memory; that is to say, they are incapable of thought and cannot participate in man's peculiarly human acts on this earth. As one Platonist argues, *all*

[29] Paraphrase of a passage in Ficino's *De divino furore* in the *Opera*, 1. 2. 614.

[30] Bowra, pp. 5-14.

man's intellect and therefore his actions depend upon the memory of past things. Within memory man finds all sensible forms, and by them he judges and acts. Through memory, then, man governs the earth and imitates the One, in whom all forms subsist.[31] But these glories do not exist for the man without heavenly fire; he has unwittingly excluded himself from the few who join the poet in developing their minds through memory and so govern the earth with judgment. One can say then that memory distinguishes the poet's proper audience, just as it had separated the poet from his false imitators and, in a different manner, the poet from the philosopher, who, though he may use memory, excludes her images from his abstract discourse. There are the few who, like the poet, recognize pure beauty and perceive the idea in the image, and there are the many who cannot.

We can see then that Platonism does not contradict any of the assumptions the allegorist made about his oral art; rather, as we shall see later, it presupposes oral conditions. It complements and deepens the ideas behind allegory while it reconciles the poet to his own failure. He need not discard his memory techniques, nor does he have to renounce his teaching role in society. In fact, he can now justify his failure by a philosophic analysis of human nature. His failure was the inevitable result of his own intentions. If he wished to create vision in others, he had to remember that few wanted to have their lives changed by vision. He could not achieve his ends except with a few people. If Orpheus in the faraway past had succeeded where the allegorist did not, Orpheus did not have the same problems. He had only to set up moral norms, he did not have to reform an already settled morality. He spoke to a people without any culture at all —at least according to the myth. He brought a moral vision to a people who had never had anything of the sort before. He literally created society. The allegorical poet, on the other hand,

31 *Asclepius* 32, in the *Corpus Hermeticum*, ed. A. D. Nock (Paris, 1945), vol. 2.

found himself cast in the role of moral reformer. His society already existed and had its own values, albeit false ones. The people of his time instinctively feared the poet's vision, for it would have required them to change their mode of thought and their moral lives. Orpheus' savage audience had no customs to change and no morality. It makes all the difference in the world whether the poet speaks to an audience at an early stage of civilization or to one at a late and decadent stage. The poet remains the same, but his audience differs radically.

Platonism likewise deepened the poet's understanding of his oral art and gave to him a new interpretation of Hesiod's old myth. To say that Zeus unites with Mnemosyne to produce the Muses is another way of saying that Zeus really is Mnemosyne. The soul finds its principle of judgment to be memory itself, as Spenser well knew; it knows what is beautiful because it recalls what is beautiful. In Plotinian terms the principle of beauty is "something that is perceived at the first glance, something which the Soul names as from an *ancient knowledge* and, *recognizing,* welcomes it, enters into unison with it."[32] The act of judgment is a memorial act.

For the modern critic, Platonism, on the contrary, does require a considerable alteration in his way of reading allegory. The modern critic is a formalist; he is accustomed to isolate for his analysis a "poem-as-object," something "out there" like a book. He turns a poem into an aesthetic object and does not see its function in society. He worries about Spenser's messy plot in Book Four of *The Faerie Queene* and wants to have Amoret reconciled to Scudamor, forgetting that Spenser may not have cared particularly about his story as an end in itself. Such a formal approach, while not wrong, is simply inadequate for an understanding of a poet like Edmund Spenser, because it ignores the rhetorical purpose of his poetry. Spenser wants to stimulate vision within another person, he wants to create a moral change

[32] *Enneads* 1. 6. 2, in the MacKenna translation. The italics are mine.

within a man's soul. If Book Four of *The Faerie Queene* succeeds in this purpose, it is a good poem, whether the story hangs together or not.

Plotinus' contention, that art surpasses its artifacts, follows necessarily from the poet's rhetorical purposes, and Spenser implies the same position in his Platonic Hymns. Spenser's lover draws out of external objects a more refined form, reduced to its first perfection. Similarly, the poet's idea or vision is the important thing; the allegory or poem has value insofar as it communicates this vision. It follows then that the critic must value poetry not for what it is but for what it stimulates—ecstasy and insight. The poet has as his task not the creation of art objects but the re-creation of vision within another person. It is not enough for an individual to regard a poem as an external spectacle in which he does not participate. If he does so, the poet has failed and provided mere entertainment. Rather, the hearer must bring the poet's vision within himself and see it as he knows himself. He must recognize that the poet's vision is his own, that the poet has revealed to him what he has always looked for in vain. Someone in ecstasy—filled with Apollo or one of the Muses— has found this strength to perceive divinity within himself.[33] As a practical consequence of this theory, one might say that a poem truly exists only when it is spoken and establishes a special kind of communication between two minds, when both recall the same vision. Such an argument once more presupposes oral conventions. The reader does not isolate for analysis a "poem-as-object." Instead he shares in vision through words. One cannot separate the listener from the poem, for his memorial act ultimately justifies the poem's existence, as the poet's memorial act causes it.

Mnemosyne obviously still meant very much to the allegorical poets and critics of the English Renaissance, steeped as they were in the ancient conventions of oral poetry and in the fashionable Platonism of the period, and she had great power among

[33] *Enneads* 5. 8. 10; Spenser's *Hymne of Beavtie*, 211-17.

their metaphysical successors too, as Louis Martz has shown in his *Poetry of Meditation* and particularly in *The Paradise Within*. Memory dominated the method of Augustinian meditation and had a crucial part in Jesuit meditations. The metaphysical poets used both forms. But the goddess could not long withstand the flood of printed material coming from the new presses. As Thamus said to Theuth about the latter's invention of letters: "This discovery of yours will create forgetfulness in the learners' souls, because they will not use their memories," a remark repeated in Alexander Dicson's *De umbra rationis* during the debate on memory in the 1580's.[34] When the Romantics revived poetry more than two centuries later, they ascribed to imagination the functions of memory. Other reasons must be given, of course, to explain so complex a change; the romantic idolization of the individual might be one. But, whatever the reasons, Memory herself had been forgotten.

Or had she? Wordsworth's famous statement: "[Poetry] takes its origin from emotion recollected in tranquillity"[35] has a suspiciously antique ring about it.

[34] *Phaedrus* 275, in the Jowett translation. For Dicson, see Yates, *Art of Memory*, pp. 268-69

[35] From the Preface to the second edition of the *Lyrical Ballads*, in the Hutchinson-Selincourt edition of the *Poetical Works* (Oxford, 1953), p. 740*a*.

❧ 5 ❧

The Auditor's Response:
The Interpretation of Allegory

WE HAVE SEEN HOW, in an extended oral-type discourse like *The Faerie Queene*, the auditor focuses his attention on specific episodes and has a general consciousness of the broad outlines of the story or plot. The characteristic modes of allegorical criticism reflect these two responses, for the exegete either discusses a particular passage or short poem in great detail and depth or elucidates the allegorical meanings of the plot as a whole, often in a very abbreviated form. It will be the purpose of this chapter to concentrate primarily on the latter operation, since it is the simpler mode, reserving the criticism of small segments for the next chapter. At the same time we will try to grasp here the main principles behind allegorical interpretation, leaving to the next chapter their application to specific texts.

I
The Principles of Interpretation

In his interpretation of plots the allegorical critic ignored a distinction normally drawn by twentieth-century critics, that between myth and the literary work conceived in its own right. Boccaccio discussed myths for thirteen books in his *Genealogy of the Gentile Gods* and then in the last two books defended his attempts by exalting the study of poetry, referring to specific works like the *Aeneid* or Petrarch's *Eclogues*. Lodge shifts from literary to myth criticism without a word to indicate the differ-

ence.[1] These critics tacitly assume that a myth like that of the
Gorgon Medusa has certain meanings contained within itself,
regardless of who adapts it. This idea corresponds precisely to
C. S. Lewis' definition of myth: "There is, then, a particular kind
of story which has a value in itself—a value independent of its
embodiment in any literary work."[2] They further assumed that
poets would naturally work with myth because its extra dimension perfectly mirrors the allegorical character of their own creations. Marlowe did not need to create elaborate meanings in the
Faust legend, because they were already there. His job was more
that of the craftsman who must arrange his material in appropriate fashion. Natalis Comes brings myth and allegory together
when he says that the only proper name which can be given to
myth criticism is allegory.[3]

Critics could identify myth and allegory because they recognized a basic kinship between them. A myth, like a metaphor or
an extended allegory, is by definition open-ended: it invites interpretation. As Lewis demonstrates, a summary of the Orpheus
myth—his descent into Hades in particular—evokes deep responses from anyone who hears it.[4] This is true of allegorical
tales as well. To take an example from Spenser: Saint George
set out from the court of the Faerie Queene to kill a dragon in
the Garden of Eden. The whole idea of reversing the Genesis
narrative of the Fall is immediately arresting and demands interpretation. Or take an old romance like that of Huon, who on a
journey from Paris to Babylon met the Fairy King Oberon in his
magical wood and there received great gifts of power. The basic
plot of an allegory must always be mythic. Where it is not, the
poet has failed—has not succeeded in converting his tale into
metaphor.

Myths and allegories are also open-ended in the literal sense

[1] Smith, 1: 65-66.
[2] *An Experiment in Criticism* (Cambridge, 1961), p. 41.
[3] *Mythologiae* 1. 5. f6ᵛ.
[4] *Experiment*, pp. 40-41.

of that term. The action of the story does not resolve itself in Aristotelian fashion but leads into another story, which is either implied by the poet or narrated later. Ovid built his whole book of *Metamorphoses* around the open-endedness of myth. The story of Phaëthon, for example, does not end with his death but leads into three other stories which depend upon his fall: the metamorphosis of his mother and sisters into trees, the transformation of his cousin into a swan, and finally one of Jove's romances in Arcady, which took place while he was investigating the extent of the disaster across the world—a story which in turn leads into another tale, that of Juno's vengeance on the nymph. Every end is another beginning, and myth never really allows a person to go away in "calm of mind all passion spent" (*Samson Agonistes* 1758). Even apocalyptic myths, where an absolute end to things is represented, end in a new beginning. After Ragnarök there will be a new earth, new gods, new men, and a new sun, and the Book of Revelation concludes with a new heaven and earth and a new city of Jerusalem descending to earth from heaven. In the same fashion, allegorical plots habitually end inconclusively. After vindicating his innocence and regaining his dukedom, Huon of Bordeaux discovers that he must journey back to the East and meet Oberon in Montmure four years hence. Oberon weeps over the sufferings he will endure, repeating the ritual action which he had done before every major episode previously. Huon is not particularly overjoyed to find that his journeys are starting all over again and remarks: "Seeing this is your pleasure, I *ought* to be well pleased therewith."[5] Likewise all of Spenser's knight-errants end their quests only to set out for new ones. In Book One, which ends more conclusively than the rest and where one would expect finality—man has regained the Garden of Eden—the Red Cross Knight must content himself with a betrothal ceremony instead of a wedding and return to Cleopolis, where he will serve Gloriana for another six years.

[5] *Huon of Bordeaux*, trans. Lord Berners and Robert Steele (London, 1895), p. 302. Italics are mine.

The great pattern for this kind of action is, of course, the *Odyssey*, where Ulysses returns after twenty years and has to tell Penelope that he must set out on yet another journey to propitiate Poseidon. One myth leads into another, and no allegorical tale ever really ends. They remain open not only to interpretation but to further stories.

In this perspective the current dispute whether *The Faerie Queene* is a whole work or a fragment loses much of its point. The wholeness which critics look for in Spenser does not exist. Even if Spenser had completed all twelve books which he promised in his Letter to Raleigh, his ending would have turned out to be the temporal beginning of the other eleven books, and the whole work itself looked forward to the future career of Arthur as a king, which itself ends in mystery, one never knowing whether Arthur died or not. No allegorical poem was ever finished in our sense of the term; and, therefore, it was quite appropriate that so many medieval and Renaissance poets should try to write immensely long poems, beyond human ability to complete. They did not absolutely need to finish them. Their plots were made up of episodes, but the plots themselves functioned in the manner of an episode: they led on to something else. An allegorical tale resembles a maze of separate rooms through which the critic picks his way, only to discover that the maze itself is part of a larger complex, which in turn is a maze. Theseus cannot escape from the Labyrinth.

In this kind of open-ended discourse the critic tries to close the poet's analogy with his own unspoken words or interpretations, but he usually learns that no one of his interpretations will suffice. If he asks one kind of question, he will get one set of answers; if another, another, and so on endlessly, at least in theory. This diversity of interpretations compounds itself the more critics there are who interpret a given work. As Boccaccio remarks in the Preface to his *Genealogy of the Gentile Gods*, "as many minds, so many opinions." These various interpretations represent the famous "levels" of allegory, referred to constantly by the critics. If a critic concerns himself with the literal content of a story, he produces a literal interpretation. If he asks moral questions, he discovers the moral allegory of a poem. But there is a limit in fact, though not in theory, to the number of levels which a critic could find in a work, for he cannot ask an infinite number of different questions. The result among critics like Golding and Harington is not the well-known four levels of biblical criticism, which are rather irrelevant to Renaissance poetry. Instead, the critics followed the old classical divisions, discussed in an earlier chapter, and talked of three main levels: the literal, moral, and allegorical. The latter category actually included a diversity of interpretations, generally involving political, cosmological, psychological, and theological levels. Thus, the formal classification included three levels, but the actual variety extended to much more than the biblical four.

Since all interpretations were considered at best partial explanations of a text, it followed that no critic need try to account for everything in an allegory. Landino has Alberti admit in the *Quaestiones Camaldulenses* that he ignored those sections of the *Aeneid* which did not fit his interpretation.[6] On the surface such a position seems to be rather a justification for slipshod criticism, but actually it corresponds to the real practice of allegorical poets. It is rather absurd to think that a poet could consciously create in every episode of his poem four or seven levels of meaning. Generally, he concentrated on one or two levels in each section, moving from one perspective to another. The critic, then, who asks one kind of question at a time, be it moral or theological, must not expect to elucidate every episode of a poem. It follows too that the principal control which the poet has over his auditors' response comes through the text of the poem itself. The most ingenious critic could not fit a cosmological interpretation to the Corceca episode in Book One of *The Faerie Queene*. He may ask moral and religio-political questions but not questions of natural philosophy. The poet can further arrange his

[6] Chastel, p. 142.

allegory so as to force his interpreters from one level to another. Dante adopts this technique in the opening canto of the *Divine Comedy*. He begins in moral allegory, when he has his pilgrim awake to the *error* of his life and try to escape from the dark wood. But by the end of the canto the type of response has been shifted. Dante the Pilgrim cannot save himself because of the Wolf, which chases him back into the wood. Virgil explains to him that the Wolf will pursue him until he kills him, but his solution to the problem of the Wolf is political, as opposed to his answer for Dante's own dilemma. A Greyhound will come to Italy and reform the government. He proposes in effect a political solution to a force which so far seemed to operate on the level of private morality. Thus, Dante forces his auditor, will he nill he, to shift levels, if he wishes to understand the symbolism of the Wolf.

The *lucus a non lucendo* principle provides a corollary to this idea of partial exegesis. The critic could conceivably reverse the meaning of an episode when he thought it necessary, for allegory could always be ironic as well as analogical. In his *Genealogy* Boccaccio applies it to the myth of the Gorgons, replacing Fulgentius' analogical understanding with an ironic one. Fulgentius thought that the Gorgons, the sight of whose faces turned men to stone, symbolized three kinds of terror, a plausible interpretation which closely follows the literal context of the story. Boccaccio reverses the literal meaning and equates the Gorgons with the unusual, startling kind of beauty which reduces men to silence (GDG 10. 10). Such an interpretation, ingenious and perverse though it may be, can at least be defended; for, as Boccaccio argues in another place, the ancients who created the myths have died long since and have left their creations "for posterity to interpret according to their own judgment" (GDG, Preface).

The critic likewise had to keep in mind that the poet, if he shifted levels on him, could change the meanings of his symbols at the same time. William Nelson in his *Poetry of Edmund*

Spenser has shown, for example, that the Night of the Mutabilitie Cantoes has no relation in *meaning* to the Night of Book
One;[7] the particular problem or theme controls the symbols, not
vice versa. This shifting symbolism obviates the modern practice of following a symbol or group of symbols through a text,
for it is getting at the problem the wrong way around. Such
symbol changes depend heavily upon the episodic nature of allegorical works. Each episode is isolated slightly from the others
and must be kept separate if the levels and symbols are not to
become hopelessly confused. Spenser deliberately breaks up not
only his narrative, as Hughes complained long ago,[8] but his
stanzas as well, bringing his story to a full stop with an Alexan-
drine every nine lines and allowing his auditors time for concentration on specific details. For the critic this practice meant that
he had to analyze a text episode by episode as Pico does in the
Heptaplus to the Genesis narrative of Creation, and he had to
shift the meanings of his symbols around. For Pico the waters
over which the Spirit hovered on the first day represent the "acci-
dental qualities and affectations of matter" (1. 2), while on the
second day they symbolize the elements which the firmament
separates into pure (the waters above the heaven) and mixed
(the waters below the heaven). He defends his procedure by
reference to the traditional practices of allegorical interpretation,
using Basil and Origen as examples (3. 4).[9]

What the poet could not or did not wish to limit were the
responses to his basic story or myth and to certain episodes which
we ourselves would call mythic. Spenser may indicate certain
levels of meaning in the Mammon episode, for example; but
Guyon's descent into hell suggests endless interpretations, just
as does Britomart's adventure in the House of Busirane or Red
Cross's battle with the Dragon. Similarly, the total plot, like a

---

[7] William Nelson, *The Poetry of Edmund Spenser* (New York, 1963),
p. 305.
[8] In *Spenser's Critics*, ed. William Mueller (Syracuse, 1959), pp. 19, 27.
[9] In Garin, p. 260.

myth, invites all levels of understanding. Harington found literal, moral, philosophical, and theological levels in the story of the Gorgon Medusa, and one could do the same with Red Cross's journey to Eden. It was, perhaps, a consciousness of this infinite openness which led Dante and Spenser to append letters of explanation to their works, for they wanted to provide some guidelines for their auditors, even if extratextual. They were journeying with the poet across uncharted seas, to use one of the most conventional metaphors for the allegorical experience. It is this limitlessness in myth particularly which makes it the most appropriate introduction to the levels of allegory. Any and all of them can be illustrated from a single story.

II
The Literal Level

Critics commonly regarded the literal level of allegory in much the way we regard fiction. It contained no truth but was a feigning. To those who attacked poetry as a form of lying, the apologists replied that the poet never pretended that his stories were true. They could not lie even if they wished to.[10] This argument, however, existed mostly for apologetic purposes. While it is true that the literal level of an allegory in its actual form does not pretend to truth, it is wrong to assume that it does not have a basis in historical fact, for the poets habitually modeled the literal level of their allegories on historical events, generally refracting the truth of specific occurrences through the distorting lens of euhemeristic myth. In the words of Plutarch, poetic myth reflects the truths of past events like a cloud, which turns the rays of the sun into a rainbow.[11] Or one can say that the poet brings up from the sea bottom the wrecks of the past and restores them to public use (the image is Cowley's in the *Muse* 36-41). In the process the past suffers "a sea-change/Into

10 For example, see Harington's argument (in Smith, 2: 201).
11 *Isis and Osiris* 20.

something rich and strange" (*Tempest* 1. 2. 400-401). The interpreter of allegory on the literal level tried to find the original events behind the myth and, therefore, wished to establish the precise relation between poetic myth and history. He did not trouble himself with form criticism as we understand it. A practical illustration of literal exegesis will explain his methods better than a theoretical discussion. In this case we will use the myth of Perseus and the Gorgon, which Boccaccio, Natalis Comes, and Harington all discussed.

In the story, as Ovid tells it, Perseus, the son of Jove, cut off the snaky head of the Gorgon Medusa, which had the power of turning men to stone. She had once had beautiful hair; but, after Neptune raped her in the Temple of Minerva, the goddess took revenge and changed her hair into serpents. Perseus cut off her head while she slept, using his bronze shield as a mirror to see her face. Boccaccio in his historical interpretation locates the Gorgon and her two sisters in the Dorcades Islands, somewhere in the Aethiopian Ocean, and makes Medusa the daughter of an actual King Phorcus, though not, as he says, the Phorcus who ruled Sardinia (*GDG* 10. 10). Medusa's enemy, Perseus, was the son of a Cretan monarch named Jupiter, who later made himself into the supreme god of the Greeks (*GDG* 12. 25).[12] In his life Perseus was a mighty hero who gave his name to the Persians and founded their capitol, Persepolis. Boccaccio uses Eusebius' account in the *Liber Temporum* to explain that Perseus looted Medusa's kingdom.[13]

Natalis Comes discusses and then rejects two different historical explanations. He knew that according to Pausanias Perseus had led an expedition from the Pelopponesus against Medusa, the daughter of King Phorcus, who ruled over the people of the Tritonian Marsh, a district south of Carthage. By a ruse

[12] Davies likewise makes Jove into a Cretan monarch in his *Orchestra*. See *Silver Poets of the Sixteenth Century*, ed. Gerald Bullett (London, 1960), p. 332. The interpretation was a familiar one.
[13] *GDG* 10. 11.

Perseus decapitated her one night in camp and carried her head back with him to Greece. In another version Medusa became a wild man from Africa who plagued the Tritonians until Perseus rescued them. Natalis rejects these two explanations not because he thinks them to be false but because they are not brilliant and useful enough in moral thought.[14]

Harington has still another explanation of the history. For him as well as for Boccaccio Perseus was the son of Jupiter, a Cretan king, but he then equates Crete with Athens, locates Medusa in the same area, and makes her into a tyrant. He tosses in an etymology of *Gorgon* which "in Greeke signifieth earth," and which appears also in Boccaccio's discussion of Demogorgon (*GDG* 1, Pro.). He then goes on to explain that Perseus' ascent to heaven in the myth represented the glorification he received from the people "for his vertuous parts."[15]

Explanations varied considerably, but everyone agreed that the myth embodied a historical sequence of events. In like manner a new poet chose for his subject either such myths or other events in history open to a euhemeristic interpretation like the wars of Charlemagne, the First Crusade, or "the historye of king Arthure" (the list and the quotation are in Spenser's Letter to Raleigh), which became respectively *Orlando Furioso, Jerusalem Delivered*, and *The Faerie Queene*.

The function of this euhemerism was twofold. On the one hand it provided a certain amount of concrete fact to the poet's fictions and supplemented the education one received in the schools, where, as Walter Ong remarks in his study of Peter Ramus, all knowledge was equated with abstract knowledge.[16] More important, it enabled the poet to exalt and debase various individuals, sometimes his own contemporaries. He could make men into gods or into beasts and leave them to be remembered

14 *Mythologiae* 7. 11.

15 Smith, 2: 202.

16 Walter J. Ong, *Ramus, Methodology and the Decay of Dialogue* (Cambridge, Mass., 1958), p. 156.

as such for all time to come. Golding so interpreted the many transformations in Ovid's *Metamorphoses* (Epistle to Leicester, 55-62). The poet was classifying people for posterity. On the positive side Spenser could transform his queen into Gloriana, enthroned in her palace at Cleopolis with its crystal tower and bridge of brass, built by magic over the "glassy See" (*FQ* 2. 10. 73). Men could become gods through the medium of poetry.

All this contrasted sharply with the original purposes of euhemerism, which began rather as a debunking movement, designed to show that the gods were really men. Now the emphasis was on the other side. If the gods were human, then men were gods. Bruno says in the *Spaccio* that, since men are celestial, "they can become gods with little effort." In another place he has Sophia say: "They did not adore Jove as if he were Divinity, but adored Divinity as it was in Jove."[17] The Florentines provided a philosophical basis for this attitude. Pico has God say to Adam in his *Oration*:[18]

> Neither heavenly nor earthly, neither mortal nor immortal have We made thee. Thou, like a judge appointed for being honorable, art the molder and maker of thyself; thou mayest sculpt thyself into whatever shape thou dost prefer. Thou canst grow downward into the lower natures which are brutes. Thou canst again grow upward from thy soul's reason into the higher natures which are divine.

In one sense the poet's eulogies were strictly fictional and complimentary, but in another sense they corresponded to the real potential inherent in any human being. Or, in other words, euhemerism derives its depth and seriousness from the higher, philosophical levels of allegory. For Spenser, Elizabeth might well in fact exist on the semidivine level, and those in bondage to Acrasia might lead an animal existence.

This euhemerism *in praxis*, though unacknowledged by the

---

[17] Giordano Bruno, *The Expulsion of the Triumphant Beast*, trans. Arthur D. Imerti (New Brunswick, N.J., 1964), pp. 266, 237-38.
[18] In Garin, pp. 104-6.

apologists, tended further to blur the traditional distinctions made by the theologians between Scripture and poetry. Boccaccio had argued for the essentially literary form of revelation,[19] and the poets tacitly assumed that their fictions had a historical basis, as did the theologians for the Bible. Moreover, the poets claimed divine inspiration for themselves, as did the theologians for scriptural writers. Amid all these similarities one distinction remained and that a crucial one. Boccaccio or Harington never contended that the events behind their stories were themselves allegorical, for they believed that the poet made allegory out of the events. There is nothing symbolic in the historical Perseus' adventure with the daughter of King Phorcus, but the poet made the story symbolic when he translated it into myth. This practice does not correspond to the scriptural *allegoria in factis*, where the departure of the Jews from Egypt has an allegorical dimension contained within the event, aside from the literary form in which it is presented. For the theologian, God alone makes poetry out of history, reflecting or anticipating one event in another. The poet could, however, imitate this divine symbolism in a human way by juxtaposing different epochs within a single fiction, as Spenser did in *The Faerie Queene* or Crashaw did in his Epiphany Ode.

In Book One Spenser complicates his euhemeristic myth by bringing together elements from four or five different periods of human history. He begins with his hero, Saint George, out on his quest to slay the dragon and rescue the Lady and her beleaguered town; that is, he starts out with the legend of a martyr who lived under Diocletian and was executed in A.D. 303. But when George falls into Orgoglio's prison, Spenser sends Prince Arthur to help him, another legendary character but this time from the sixth century. Things become still more confused at the end, when George meets his dragon not in Libya but in the Garden of Eden and redoes the story of the Fall—backward. Instead of going from innocence to sin through the wiles of the

[19] GDG 14. 9.

serpent, the formerly sinful George kills the dragon and liberates the land, cleansing it from evil. This is, of course, an allegory of Christian salvation, but on the historical level it seems as if Spenser were unsatisfied with the actual events of the past and were doing them over again, only in a peculiar fashion. He reverses the process of history and makes its end (the Fall) into a beginning and the beginning (Paradise) into an end. He is not peculiar in this, for Dante has his pilgrim pass from the dark wood of sin through hell and purgatory back to the Garden of Eden, where human history began and where his purification is completed. In Spenser this technique becomes still more complicated when we remember the apocalyptic symbolism of Book One. The dragon is also the Ancient Serpent, defeated at the end of time, and Spenser seems to be suggesting that the Apocalypse really involves a reversal of the pattern of events with which history began. The Beginning becomes the End, just as in the whole epic the last book is the temporal beginning. To add further confusion, the political allegory of the poem brings in Queen Elizabeth and the whole intricate world of Armada politics. Spenser has done much more than mythologize a particular historical event, for he has jumbled together characters and situations from all over human history and unified them within a single narrative. The effect has meaning, as we shall see when we discuss the moral level of allegory, but it depends upon a divine perspective on human history, where all the happenings in time are simultaneously present and can be seen to manifest an ordered pattern.

A natural example might help us to familiarize ourselves more with this peculiar kind of history; for every night, when a person looks at the stars, he sees the same kind of jumble. The light from the stars takes many years to come to the earth and consequently represents their past rather than their present condition. Or, more accurately, the human spectator experiences a confusion of different historical periods, for he sees some stars as they were eight years ago and others as they were 180,000 years ago. Despite this historical confusion he does perceive an ordered pattern; one which exists only from a human perspective, but one which has special human significance. Men have sailed by the stars and have found their own fate in the astral patterns of the night sky. The old seers of Chaldea and Rome failed to realize that they were seeing not their own but the stars' fate. What had already happened to the stars became a present actuality for man, seen from endless, remote distances. Similarly, in *The Faerie Queene* the auditor sees as a present reality the careers of Saint George, Arthur, and Queen Elizabeth, all of whom he knows lived at different times, but he recognizes in this series of juxtapositions a pattern of meaning. He sees something like that which the Divine Mind would see and with some of the remoteness of a Godlike perspective or of a human being looking at the stars. Spenser accentuates this sense of distance by his ceremonial language and archaic words, which never allow the auditor to forget that what he is hearing happened a long time ago and which give to his experience a sense of immense distances. To use Keats's description, Spenser's romance is a "Queen of far-away" who melodizes in her "olden pages" ("On Sitting Down to Read *King Lear* Once Again").

Crashaw achieves a similar medley of historical periods in his hymn *In the Gloriovs Epiphanie of Ovr Lord God*, long known for its brilliant philosophical mysticism. He begins the poem where one would expect him to start—with the song of the Three Kings who have just arrived in Bethlehem from Persia. In the middle he shifts through prophecy to the Crucifixion, thirty years later. So far the juxtaposition is simple and quite natural, since the Epiphany and Birth of Christ derive their significance from the sacrifice on the Cross; but, when analyzed more carefully, the hymn reveals another historical dimension. The Kings devote much of the hymn to an attack on sun worship and its related deities: Mithra, Isis, and Osiris. Their polemic calls to mind the great struggle between Christianity and the mystery religions in the third century, which reached a kind of climax when the Emperor Aurelian established the cult of Sol Invictus on the Quirinal Hill.[20] The festival of the sun occurred at the winter solstice, and the Christians countered it by celebrating the birthday of Christ, the true sun, born in the darkness of the night. Crashaw's hymn thus includes at least three historical events: the coming of the wise men from the east, the death of Christ, and the triumph of Christianity over the heliolatry of the Roman Empire. It may include still a fourth, this one a contemporary event. Crashaw stayed with the Royalist exiles in Paris, and it was shortly before this time that Tommaso Campanella had proclaimed Louis XIV the monarch who would unite all peoples in a new city of the sun and be himself the new Sun King.[21] For Crashaw no sun, particularly one established by the state, can be allowed to obscure the true sun, Jesus Christ.

The process of euhemeristic myth-making is extraordinarily complex, but its purpose remains clear. When the poet runs together different periods of history and exalts or debases his characters beyond the human level, he is imitating divine judgment, seeing history from a point of view outside time and passing moral judgment on certain individuals. One cannot present Queen Elizabeth as Gloriana or Mary Stuart as the witch Duessa without a very definite moral perspective. The poet judges people by what they make of themselves, and in this sense he shares in Pico's philosophical outlook. Man is what he becomes, whether it be a rational human being, a vegetable, or an angel. The poet's images define the result. In this sense euhemeristic myth is always moral history and, hence, demands a moral level of allegory. The one presupposes the other.

[20] See Gibbon, *The Decline and Fall of the Roman Empire* (New York, n.d.), 1: 271; and Franz Cumont, *The Oriental Religions in Roman Paganism* (New York, 1956), pp. 114-15.
[21] Yates, GB, pp. 361, 390-91.

III
The Moral Level

When someone looks for the moral vision behind the clouds of historical myth, he must suffer intense disappointment, especially if he is using a critic like Boccaccio, Hawes, or Golding. Boccaccio, for example, takes the story of Medusa's rape by Neptune and reduces it to the level of the Book of Proverbs. Neptune's love for Medusa's golden hair signifies his love of money. Their love-making in Minerva's Temple becomes a prudential marriage; the transformation of Medusa's hair into snakes indicates the unending cares caused by the possession of wealth; and the beheading, the loss of goods by which a man lives and has power (GDG 10. 11). None can deny the ingeniousness of this interpretation, but it hardly betrays any brilliance in moral thought. Natalis Comes equals Boccaccio in this combination of ingenuity and triviality. For him Medusa symbolizes either the power of pleasure, which makes people useless (turns them to stone), or, if one concentrates on the transformation of her hair, the kind of person who glories in his own talent and despises God, for which attitude he loses his talent and receives a bad one in its place. Harington has another dull version, expressed in more general terms:[22]

> Morally it signifieth this much: *Perseus* a wise man, sonne of Iupiter, endewed with vertue from aboue, slayeth sinne and vice, a thing base & earthly signified by Gorgon, and so mounteth vp to the skie of vertue.

These exegeses may well surprise us, since one would hardly think that a rape symbolized a *marriage de convenance*, but the disappointment remains. The poet's morality seems distressingly commonplace.

[22] *Mythologiae* 7. 11; Smith, 2: 202.

Golding's version of Ovid depresses one still more, for it generally lacks even ingenuity. An exception is the Narcissus myth, where he does achieve some of Boccaccio's brilliant perversity, for he says that Echo signifies the "lewd behaviour of a bawd" (Epistle to Leicester, 108). It takes some genius to misconstrue Echo in this fashion, but elsewhere Golding elaborates obvious commonplaces without this rather dubious talent. His long catalog of moral explanations soon bores one. Plotinus, on the contrary, had seen in the Narcissus myth a profound meaning. The youth symbolized for him all those bound to the phenomenological world, an interpretation both moral and psychological (*Enneads* 1. 6. 8). Renaissance critics like Golding seem to think that moral allegory necessarily lacks any depth. Or rather, moral criticism makes clichés in the expression of its own insights, but the poetry itself must depend upon more than this. Otherwise, the greatest allegories of the English Renaissance sound hollow at the core, for Spenser and others designed their poems primarily for moral purposes.

To appreciate moral allegory one must separate the experience it provides from the moral conclusions which the auditor draws from that experience and applies to particular historical contexts, his own or others, private or public. It depends, therefore, on the literal level of the poem, on the history understood euhemeristically. The poet experiences a particular event like Perseus' raid in the Dorcades and then expresses this event in terms of value. He shapes fact into myth to register his judgment of the fact. Hawes' Lady Rhetoric characterizes this method by an example:

> And also Pluto/somtyme kynge of hell
> A Cyte of Grece/standynge in thessayle
> Betwene grete rockes/as the boke doth tell
> Wherin were people/without ony fayle
> Huge/fyerse/and stronge in batayle
> Tyrauntes/theues/replete with treason

Wherfore poetes/by true comparyson

. . . .

Vnto the deuylles/blacke and tedyous
Dyde them resemble/in terryble fygure
For theyr mysse lyuynge/so foule and vycyous

[*Pastime* 1002-11]

The auditor in turn suddenly understands a particular situation prophetically; he sees it "in terryble fygure"—under judgment. He discovers that history can be conceived of mythically and that general values can be equated with certain particulars. He then explains this revelation on two levels: as fact and as value, the historical and moral levels of allegory. Hence the clichés of moral interpretation, for they express only one side of the auditor's experience. They must not be allowed to conceal the vitality of moral allegory, for the stories of the poet can guide and change a person's way of life. The man who has suddenly found hell next door cannot continue to live in quite the same fashion as before.

Within society moral allegory provided a necessary ethical education. Ong has shown that the universities hardly taught ethics at all,[23] and we have already seen that the poets considered contemporary society to be almost totally corrupt and desperately in need of moral reform. The poet did not adopt the abstract argumentation common in later periods for this purpose but tried to lift his auditors into a different thought-mode, where moral judgment became automatic. He unified fact and value through myth and wanted his auditors to think in the same way. In Aristotle's phrase, he expressed the universal through the particular and thus transcended ordinary history. In our terms he approached the modes of prophetic rhetoric. Intensely concerned with historical facts, he charged them with moral value and wished to induce a conversion or soul-change in his auditors. He knew that, once they thought like him, they could not avoid a

23 *Ramus*, pp. 140-42.

certain ethical maturity. The prophet asked for an immediate decision; the poet, for a new kind of sensibility, from which such decisions could come.

As a result of this thought control, the auditor imitated the mythic figures of the poet and used them for models. Sidney alludes to this when he argues that the poet's special task is "to bestow a *Cyrus* upon the world to make many *Cyrusses.*"[24] The real Cyrus never had all the ideal qualities which Xenophon gave to his mythical Cyrus and, therefore, had less of reality to him, if continuing influence signifies a kind of vitality which escapes the laws of mortality and consequently participates in a kind of Platonic truth. The poet created in his allegories enduring models for society to follow. It was not his business to mirror society or human nature as it existed, but to create better, more ideal forms of them. In his case the old principle had to be reversed: art did not imitate nature; nature imitated art.

There can be no doubt of the utility and peculiar power in moral allegory, but by itself it remains insufficient. It cannot explain why the poets insisted on veiling truth, and, as we have seen, it is this concealment of truth which alone defines the special mode of allegorical rhetoric. In his indictment of contemporary poetry Reynolds made precisely this point.[25] He accused the poets of veiling the obvious, and there is certainly nothing in the critical statements and clichés produced by moral allegory which need be hidden. Boccaccio might think that prudential marriages were evil, but he could not argue that this fact had to be concealed from the multitude. There were truths which the poet wanted to veil, but these did not exist on the literal and moral levels of his art. One found them rather in the various allegorical levels of the poem properly so called, which Harington lists as political, philosophical, and theological.

[24] *Defence of Poesie,* in Feuillerat's edition of the *Prose Works* (Cambridge, 1963), 3: 8. Hereafter referred to as *Defence,* F3.
[25] Spingarn, 1: 164.

IV
The Allegorical Levels
The Political Level

The political level of allegory presents a special case among the inner core of meanings known to the critics. It stands out because the truth which the poet conceals has no inherent need for the veil but rather depends upon external circumstances. In the Renaissance as in the twentieth century the writer sometimes felt constrained to maintain political positions unpopular with those in power, and he shielded himself from censure by a deliberate obscurantism. Spenser made the political allegory of his *Shepheardes Calender* so obscure that no one has satisfactorily explained it yet, and his own contemporaries were confused.[26] Even so, he did not always escape censure. Burleigh suppressed one of his volumes for what he considered to be personal attacks upon himself, and King James of Scotland protested publicly over Spenser's treatment of his mother in *The Faerie Queene*.[27] Spenser may have been fortunate to die before James inherited the English throne. The poet could not avoid veiling what he said anymore than he could avoid saying it. Spenser in particular regarded with intense interest the political issues of his own day and wished to present his own attitude to them in his allegories. But, if he wanted his books to be published or wished to retain his livelihood, he had to be careful. Hence, the veil.

The actual technique of political allegory differs little from that of euhemeristic myth. An example from Boccaccio will manifest this similiarity. In his *Sixth Eclogue* he wished to celebrate the return of Giovanna and her husband, Louis of Taranto, to Naples. They had been driven from their realm by King Louis of Hungary, who later had been forced to withdraw his armies, en-

[26] See Webbe's comment in Smith, 1: 264.
[27] Nelson, pp. 8, 13-16.

abling the two to return. For this occasion Boccaccio adapted Virgil's myth of the golden age returned, which the Roman poet had used for the same purpose—to proclaim a political position. The eclogue begins with Meliboeus mourning for the exiled Alcestus (Louis of Taranto), though it is a festival day. Amintas comes and tells him the good news: Poliphemus (the Hungarian King) has retired and Alcestus has actually returned. In joy the two shepherds sing the Virgilian hymn of the new golden age, while the altars fume, the flocks graze, and the fields remain in quiet peace. Alcestus has brought back with him Astraea and has united the wolf and the flock in common toil.

In this eclogue Boccaccio mythologizes the present in the same way that Spenser did the age of King Arthur. The specific events of history take on the larger splendor of myth. The only difference between the two levels is temporal: one reflects the past, the other, the present. In more complex allegories the two levels often were combined in the same myth. Spenser's tale of Arthur mirrors both past and present. Arthurian history already existed as euhemeristic myth and, therefore, as value. By applying this particular myth to another period of history, Spenser creates a second level of value. All he leaves for his auditor to do is to relate the old myth to new particulars, an attempt which requires considerable background in contemporary politics for a modern and may become quite difficult when the poet is being deliberately obscure. Boccaccio's eclogue does not explain itself within the text; the critic must know about Neapolitan affairs in the 1340's before he can ever interpret it properly. The modern reader of political allegory looks to his footnotes.

The trouble with political allegory is that it soon loses its effectiveness. The hidden secret of 1590 may need no concealment and may have become irrelevant by 1620 and certainly by 1960. The more contemporary a poet makes his political allegory, the less interesting it becomes for succeeding generations. No one reads Boccaccio's *Sixth Eclogue* today, and the most ardent Spenserians ignore the Fifth Book of *The Faerie Queene*, his supreme example of political allegory. A poet can escape this fate, however, if he sticks close to his myth and does not particularize his allegory too much. Virgil's *Fourth Eclogue* served a political purpose in the days of the Second Triumvirate and yet has charmed people for two thousand years. He achieved this immortality by speaking in large mythic images, which could apply to any auspicious beginning in political history and have been so adapted countless times since, as in Boccaccio's *Sixth Eclogue*. Spenser and Boccaccio failed in their political allegory because they related their images so closely to contemporary situations that they could never be applied to any similar situations. The problems of Belge died with Queen Elizabeth and could not concern later generations, while the myth of the golden age might yet be realized.

The Philosophical Levels

The cosmological and psychological levels, or what Harington would call the levels of natural philosophy, justify by themselves the veil which the poet places before truth and, therefore, the peculiar rhetorical mode of allegory. They alone explain the poet's need for concealment because, unlike the lower levels of allegory, they arise from a theory of poetic truth and not from a study of the mythic forms which it requires. On the lower levels of allegory the critic derived his ideas from the contrast which he observed between historical fact and the mythic forms which it took. In higher allegory the critic passed behind the forms to the truths which caused this distortion of fact in the first place. We have already discussed how the critics generally assumed that the poet received his truth under divine inspiration. Since this truth came to him from above, the poet could not express it simply, for he realized that it transcended the ordinary forms of human thought. As in Sallustius' time, theorists construed the content of this revelation to be a knowledge of the cosmos, its gods, and its equivalents in the human soul, so that one discovers divine truth invariably on the philosophical and theological levels of allegory.[28] Even Puttenham, who largely ignores allegorical theory, repeated the old commonplace that the early poets, from an observation of the stars, discovered the gods and invented religion. He implies that they instituted sacrifices to the gods under a delusion, but allegorical thinkers took the notion much more seriously. Ficino equated the old gods of pagan myth with the angels of the Christian tradition and defined myth as the language of the gods; Reynolds claimed that the cosmos itself afforded the fittest matter for poetry and had been the subject of the ancient fables. Everyone tended to associate the origins of poetry with sacral revelation. Even Boccaccio, who ignores cosmological speculation in his discussion of the Gorgon myth, assumes the sacral character of early poetry in the various theories about it which he criticizes.[29] Poetry had divine beginnings, and these revelations depended upon cosmic theory.

For the Florentines one can say that the cosmos literally inspired all poetry. Ficino and Pico thought of the Muses as spirits who operated the celestial world. Calliope was the *anima mundi*, and the other Muses the heavenly orbs.[30] They did not exist within the planets, as human souls inhabit bodies, but controlled them from without. Sitting upon these celestial bodies, they contemplated the invisible world within the eternal Mind[31] and imparted their simultaneous vision of the visible and invisible worlds to the poet, who could receive their inspiration because he shared in their essential nature. His own mind had once inhabited these same spheres.

He was especially adapted for his task because, as a human being, his nature mirrored all three worlds: the earth, the heavens, and the invisible world. In the *Heptaplus* Pico says, "Man

[28] *Concerning the Gods* 4; Chastel, p. 138.
[29] *Arte* 1. 3; Chastel, p. 138; Sears Jayne, *John Colet and Marsilio Ficino* (Oxford, 1963), p. 71; Spingarn, 1: 167; and *GDG* 14. 8.
[30] *De divino furore* in *Opera omnia* 1. 2. 612f; Pico della Mirandola, *A Treatise on Platonick Love*, trans. Thomas Stanley (1651), ed. Edmund Gardner (Boston, 1914), 1. 10.
[31] Ficino, *Opera omnia* 1. 2. 612.

is not so much a fourth world, like some new creature, as he is the bond and union of the three already described" (*Hep.* 5. 6).[32] Consequently, cosmological interpretation precedes psychological, for the latter needs the former for its very definition. In his commentary to Benivieni's *Sonnet*, Pico prefaces his discussion of human love with a description of the cosmos, and in the *Heptaplus* the cosmological level comes before and helps to explain the psychological level of the allegory. Bruno created a cosmic allegory in the *Spaccio*, which he intended to be understood psychologically. The two levels go together, and Spenser through all his career associated them closely. His shepherds find cosmic correspondences for their internal conditions, as does the poet himself for his wedding in the *Epithalamion*.

It follows from these principles that allegory is the essential human speech because it alone expresses human nature. Man mirrors the cosmos, and allegory automatically reveals cosmic relationships, particularly in its combination of the two *lógoi*, the invisible and visible words which imitate that combination of appearance and invisible power which make up the cosmos and the human being. Reynolds and Harington, when they complained that the loss of allegorical instruction caused a decline in the human race, presupposed this idea.[33] If man's nature consists in a union of other natures, the proper speech to express this essence will be allegory, the language which in single symbols unites the various natures of the cosmos. At the same time man proclaims by this speech his affinity and love for the external worlds. Syllogistic discourse, on the other hand, destroys this relational language by narrowing symbols to single meanings. As a result, man loses his peculiarly human speech and becomes alienated from the other worlds. Reynolds would have known from his master, Pico, that this alienation means moral decay (*Hep.* 5. 7); the harmony has been broken.[34]

32 In Garin, p. 300.
33 Smith, 2: 203-4; Spingarn, 1: 144-45.
34 In Garin, pp. 304-8.

In the actual explication of these levels the Renaissance critic used the techniques of the late classical critics. Harington discovers two interpretations of the Gorgon myth which are closely associated. In one, Perseus' struggle with Medusa signifies the battle between man's divine mind and his earthly nature. Victory allows his mind to understand or ascend to the contemplation of eternal truths, "in which contemplacion consisteth the perfection of man."[35] Harington calls this a natural allegory; Sallustius would have called it psychological. The second interpretation is cosmic and corresponds to the Attis interpretations of Julian and Sallustius. The heavenly nature (Perseus) causes motion and corruption in inferior bodies but at last severs itself from earthly things and flies up on high, where it remains forever.

To take another example, Golding finds three levels of natural philosophy in Ovid's *Metamorphoses*: two cosmological and one psychic. On the first level he sees in the many transformations which Ovid describes a symbolic representation of the old classical principle that "nothing under heaven dooth ay in stedfast state remayne" (Epistle to Leicester, 10). The sisters of Phaëthon, for instance, could not maintain their human forms, and Narcissus became a flower. This interpretation in turn suggests a corollary principle, namely "that nothing perisheth" (Epistle, 11). Matter may change its forms, but it can never cease to exist as matter. The material substance of Narcissus changed its shape, when he turned into a flower, but it remained a material substance. The psychological level relates to the two cosmological levels as the exception to the general rule. The human soul is the one thing which does remain itself and escapes death to face reward and punishment in the afterlife. The classical Hades and Elysian Fields symbolize the Christian hell and heaven. As evidence for this position, Golding cites the ancient practice of euhemeristic myth, in which noble men were made divine by the heathens for their virtues. He contends that such myth-making presupposes the immortality of the soul. This is an interesting argument because it highlights the relation between

[35] Smith, 2: 202.

the lower and higher levels of allegory. The seriousness of euhemeristic myth comes from the philosophical levels of allegory. We
have already seen that transformations in allegory could be explained by Pico's philosophical view of human nature. Golding
provides a different rationale, but in both cases the principles
behind euhemeristic myth are assumed to exist on the cosmological and psychological levels. Without this inner core, Spenser's divinization of Queen Elizabeth degenerates into empty
praise. With it his euhemerism gains a profundity it could never
have by itself. In a similar manner Golding derives his moral
level from ideas like Pico's. Man makes his own nature through
history, be it divine, human, or subhuman. A poet like Ovid
passes judgment on a person's life by the transformations he ar-
ranges for that person. Phaëthon's sisters lived a vegetable existence. This is the moral level of allegory which Golding finds in
the *Metamorphoses,* but it makes no sense without the philosophical levels. In other words, cosmological and psychological interpretation tries to explain why myths are important as well as
what they represent.

Outside myth in literary works proper, cosmological theory
could be used to characterize the total art work. A poem was assumed to imitate the world, and it became another world unto
itself. The poet tried to create the illusion of a richness and variety in his poetry which could rival that of the cosmos itself, an
attempt which C. S. Lewis says came from the old confusion of
poetry with encyclopedias.[36] For such purposes the epic poem
served especially well, with its greater length and tradition of
encyclopedic criticism. Homer was the Emperor of all wisdom,
and Virgil in the *Aeneid* "omnem humanae vitae genus ex-
primit," that is, civil law, political history, the secrets of the
cosmos, and the like.[37] Palingenius in his *Zodiake of Life* promised to write of whatever came into his mind, like a ship blown by

[36] *English Literature in the Sixteenth Century Excluding Drama* (Oxford, 1962), p. 321.
[37] For Homer see the Chapman selection in Smith, 2: 296; for Virgil
see Landino's Prooemium to his edition of the *Opera* (Strasbourg, 1502).

the wind of inspiration.[38] This principle once more depended upon extratextual assumptions. Critics thought that great writers like Homer or Moses knew everything and proceeded to find everything in their narratives, even when it meant arranging the poet's symbols in an arbitrary fashion. Before he discusses each level of Genesis, Pico carefully describes the necessary philosophical background; that is, he determines the meaning before he interprets the text. In one place he practically admits that the criticism is really his own creation. In the Proem to the Seventh Book he slips into the magisterial *we* and then corrects himself and gives the credit to Moses: "*we* have discussed . . . it remains for *us* . . . to treat . . . of the creatures whose nature *we* established in the preceding treatises; or, to speak more accurately, it remains for us to listen to Moses speaking. . . ."[39]

This technique violates our own standards of interpretation, for the critic, instead of giving himself over to the art work, fits it into his own system of thought. Not that we do not fall into the same practice on occasion. When someone asserts that Shakespeare's witches are only psychological emanations of Macbeth's character, he ignores their blatant independent existence in the play and is really arguing that Shakespeare would never treat witches and spirits in a serious manner, despite the common Renaissance belief in them. The conception of the poet determines the content of the poem and sets up standards for the critic. If the poet knows everything, as in cosmological poetry, it follows that a good critic should have a similar breadth of wisdom. Boccaccio has a long list of subjects for his poet to master, and a modern student should presumably know the same disciplines: cosmology, rhetoric, and grammar, moral and natural philosophy, astronomy, history, and geography (GDG 14. 7).

The technique of this cosmic criticism had its own rigid control, namely, the philosophical system of the critic. In Pico's

[38] *Zodiake of Life,* trans. Barnabe Googe, ed. Rosemond Tuve (New York, 1947), p. 2.
[39] In Garin, p. 324.

case this control corresponds to the one used by the wise in classical antiquity—a common theory of the cosmos. Though we may think such criticism arbitrary, Pico would argue that he had proved its validity by making the text reveal his cosmological suppositions. In two places (*Hep.* 2. Pro; 4. Pro.) he flatly states that his interpretation proves that Moses knew everything about the cosmos and human nature.[40] From our point of view any text could be turned into cosmic allegory by this technique, but the theory does affect *in fact* those poems written under its influence, like *The Shepheardes Calender* or the Platonic Hymns, which we will analyze in the next chapter. For our immediate purposes Pico's commentary on Genesis will suffice, for the *Heptaplus* provides the most extraordinary example of cosmic criticism in the Renaissance.

Pico analyzes seven levels of allegory in the opening chapter of Genesis. The first three are cosmological, the fourth is psychological, the fifth and sixth involve both levels, and the last is theological. He follows roughly the order which Harington and Golding later used, for the levels of natural philosophy lead into theology. To give some idea of the breadth and variety of his criticism, it will be enough to follow through his successive interpretations of one incident in the Priestly Narrative: the separation of the waters.

> And God said, "Let there be a firmament in the midst of the waters, and let it divide the waters from the waters." And God made the firmament, and divided the waters which were under the firmament from the waters which were above the firmament: and it was so. And God called the firmament Heaven. And the evening and the morning were the second day.
>
> [Gen. 1: 6-8]

On the first level Pico identifies the waters with the elements, which exist pure and unmixed above the region of the air and completely mixed below this region. The firmament represents

[40] Ibid., pp. 222, 266-68.

the airy middle region, where the elements exist in imperfect mixtures and appear as "rain, snow, lightning, thunder, comets, and the like" (*Hep.* 1. 3).[41] On the second level the firmament is the sphere of fixed stars which divides the empyrean from the planetary spheres, or the waters above from the waters below. On the third level the waters above the firmament signify the upper ranks of angels; the firmament, the middle ranks; and the waters below, the lower ranks. In these levels he has gone from the sublunary through the celestial to the supercelestial or invisible world. The fourth level is concerned with man, the bond and union of the three worlds. The waters above are the angelic intelligence in man, over which the Spirit broods; the firmament is equated with reason, and the waters below with man's sensory powers. In the fifth level Pico tries to show how the order of Moses' narrative paralleled the order of the cosmos. Here the firmament represents the heavens and thus has almost a literal meaning, though the waters are again symbolic. They signify the worlds of intelligible and sensible forms. For his sixth level Pico discusses the kinds of relationships possible within the cosmos and finds three different understandings of this particular episode. In one perspective the firmament and the waters represent two kinds of part-to-whole relationships: inseparable and separable. The stars are inseparable parts of the firmament, but water can always be separated from a larger body of water (6. 3). In another perspective the firmament symbolizes the Aristotelian doctrine of the mean, separating the extremes or waters from each other (6. 4). This interpretation has an additional, theological application. It implies the familiar Neoplatonic idea that the extremes can communicate only through a mean or intermediary, which shares in both natures. Christ, the God-man, unites the two extremes of man and divinity and makes it possible for them to approach each other (6. 7). Finally, Pico finds a seventh or theological level, where the episode describes a period in

[41] Ibid., p. 214. The relevant chapters in the *Heptaplus* are 1. 3; 2. 3; 3. 3; 4. 1-2; 5. 1-2; 6. 3-4, 7; 7. 2.

salvation history. The firmament signifies the Law, which separated Jew from gentile. The Jews worshipped only Yahweh, while
the gentiles paid homage to the stars; so the two are aptly symbolized by the waters *above* the firmament or sphere of fixed
stars and those *below*. In all these identifications Pico displays
a brilliant ingenuity, finding apt reasons for the wildest interpretations and displaying remarkable insight. Although we may not
approve of this kind of criticism, it has a great social utility, for
it allows a specific text to absorb within itself all the basic ideas
of a particular civilization and thus remain relevant from one age
to another. It likewise accustoms people to translating their abstract thoughts into concrete symbols. Concepts like part and
whole or mean and extreme appeal solely to man's rational powers and make no impression upon his imagination or memory;
but, when combined with the precise picture of the waters and
the firmament, they can remain long in the mind and affect more
than one power in the human psyche.

From a modern viewpoint three aspects of philosophical allegory arrest one's attention. First, the technique seems to be
extraordinarily complex and subtle. The actual levels range anywhere from two to six, and the facility with which the critics
treat the details in a narrative or myth astonishes a modern ob-
server. The second aspect, however, strikes a more radical note.
This type of criticism depends upon extratextual assumptions
about the poet's knowledge and the kind of truth he receives
under divine inspiration. No elements in the Gorgon myth itself
require this kind of interpretation; rather, the concept of the poet
determines the understanding of the poem. The literal and moral
levels had arisen from formal considerations. The mythic mode
was compared to the historical facts behind the myth, and the
comparison suggested certain exegetical principles. But in the
inner core of allegory the critic moves through the art work back
to the poet himself, trying to understand the truths behind the
myths which require this kind of rhetorical mode. In other words,
the critic passes from the veil to the truth behind the veil, from

the lower to the higher levels of allegory. The third aspect of this level, though less radical, has an appealing and nostalgic attraction for us. This kind of criticism rests upon an ancient belief, sophisticated in form but primitive in its origins, that man exists in harmony with his world. Man the microcosm shares in the same natures which make up the cosmos. What he says or thinks provokes correspondences throughout the universe, and the poet in particular creates a discourse, the symbols of which have objective correlatives in the real world. The poet does not think that he is shut up in the realm of his own mind, nor does he feel alienated from the natural world. Rather, he expresses its essence and his own qualities whenever he chooses the allegorical mode of speech. He may feel himself isolated from his own society but never from the world. Nature had not yet shrunk into a machine but was filled with mystery, and man himself was the mystery of mysteries.

The Theological Level

On the theological level the Renaissance critics differed most from their classical predecessors. Sallustius had envisaged such a level for myth, but he would never have found there what Harington or Pico did. On the Gorgon myth, for example, Harington provides a theological explanation which Sallustius would have classed as psychic. Perseus symbolizes the angelic nature, child of the most high God, which kills and destroys all bodily substance (the Gorgon) and ascends to heaven. This interpretation, with a few shifts in emphasis (from mind to nature), repeats his psychological explanation of the myth and could easily fit into Neoplatonic descriptions of the ladder. Sallustius would probably not have objected to this interpretation, but he would never have called it theological because he restricted this level to a consideration of the gods themselves and left man out.[42]

The reason for this change may have been Christianity, with

[42] Smith, 2: 202-3; *Concerning the Gods* 4.

its continual stress on the interaction of God and man through history. In fact, the most characteristic subject for theological allegory was roughly similar to the allegorical or typological level of biblical exegesis. Pico interpreted the Creation narrative as an allegory of salvation history, which in his case is not surprising, since he is working with sacred Scripture, but in another sense is surprising because he is applying the modes of classical, not biblical, allegory to his text. Golding does the same thing with Ovid. He read the stories of the Roman poet as mythic analogues to the facts of biblical history, understood typologically in the Christian tradition. Thus, Prometheus, who invented images and made man out of clay, becomes a type of the Logos, through whom Adam was made from slime in the image of God (Epistle, 434-54). In his *Eleventh Eclogue*, the *Pantheon*, Boccaccio develops the most complicated form of this typological allegory. Glaucus narrates the whole of salvation history from the Creation to the Descent of the Holy Ghost, all presented in the guise of classical myth. The Annunciation, for example, becomes the story of Mercury and Danae; the harrowing of hell, Hercules' expedition to recover the herds stolen by Cacus; the Resurrection, the myth of Hippolytus' return from the dead. In places the allegory grates uncomfortably. Acorns replace the Eucharist at the Last Supper. Nevertheless, the technique works and is based upon a genuine correspondence between the literary forms of biblical history and classical myth. Origen long before had pointed out the mythical character of such stories as the Fall and the Temptation in the Desert (*Periarchon* 4. 3. 1), but Renaissance critics were more reticent about this, perhaps because of Augustinian influence. The biblical myths were historical events to which God had added an allegorical dimension, while the classical tales were thought to be mere mirror images or distortions of these happenings. They were shadows, man's imitations of God's historical poetry.

This typological allegory degenerated when poets substituted decorative fictions for genuine myths. Antonio Geraldini provides a good example of this misused allegory. He was a minor writer of the fifteenth century who produced some eclogues based on the life of Christ, which he intended for school children. Actually, he simply retold the Gospel narrative and replaced the names and phrases of the Vulgate with classical ones. Thus, in the *Eighth Eclogue* Aegle goes to the tomb, finds the stone rolled away and two angels waiting. She then encounters Acanthus, who tells her of his resurrection and warns her not to touch him until he ascends Olympus. Change the names and you have the Johannine story of Mary Magdalene at the tomb. In this kind of allegory no real theological level exists because the classical myth has become too attenuated to stand by itself. Instead, the salvation history becomes the literal level of the allegory, hardly disguised by a classical nomenclature.

Events in salvation history did on occasion function successfully on the literal level, suggesting a different range of meanings on a theological level. Crashaw, in his Epiphany Hymn, combined a literal narrative taken from the Gospels with a refined christological mysticism. The constant, brilliant paradoxes of the poem rest upon a simple opposition, which, once grasped, clarifies practically all the difficult passages. Day represents theological and moral darkness; and darkness, light. Starting with this reversal of symbols, Crashaw merely plays variations upon the theme, as he develops its historical basis in the narrative. Misled by the beauty of light and the brightness of the world, man worshipped the sun and fell into an interior, moral darkness, from which Christ rescued him. He came by night, and at his death the sun went into a preternatural eclipse. This unusual darkness opened the eyes of men to the true light within themselves. They learned to shut their eyes, so they might see. This theological vision gives to the poem its paradoxes and makes it unique among Crashaw's works. He deserves high praise for combining the sophisticated literal history which we discussed earlier with a brilliant theology as well as with the philosophical mysticism of Dionysius the Areopagite. The poem functions on all levels.

Theological allegory obviously could assume quite diverse forms. It might appear as disguised salvation history, Christianized Neoplatonism, or theology in the true sense of the term. It capped the other levels of allegory and gave the radiance of divine truth to the poet's myth.

V
Conclusion

The evident complexity and variety of allegorical exegesis affords excellent evidence for the practical purposes served by this kind of poetry in the Renaissance. The poet was an educator, and from his myths a person could gain or reinforce an understanding of history, ethics, politics, natural philosophy, and theology. The ordinary man found entertainment in the poet's stories, and learned a little history and even some morality, to the extent that he entered into the thought-modes of euhemeristic myth. The more intelligent auditor could pass from the veil to the truths concealed behind it and find there the secrets of the cosmos, of the human soul, and of divine action. In this fashion allegory carried on the Homeric tradition, and the Renaissance poet continued to civilize his contemporaries. With such practical ends in mind, he never considered beauty or aesthetic appreciation more than a lure to draw his auditors into his classroom. Or, more accurately, he thought of beauty in a Platonic fashion and identified it with truth. In this sense his practical ends became identified with what we would call his aesthetic ends. The approach to truth was the way to beauty.

Unfortunately, his time was running out. Homer's poetry had provided the basis for education in Greece, but now a student could learn the inner secrets of poetry in the universities. The historical-moral world of euhemeristic myth still had a relevance, and it is not surprising that the avant-garde of the new age, Sidney and Jonson, reduced the ends of poetry for the most part to moral instruction. Theology and natural philosophy were no longer needed. The veil had been rent.

This breakdown of allegorical rhetoric also had tragic consequences, for it is a fact that myths can explain the inner problems of human experience in a way that discursive reason cannot.
For example, the problem of free will and determinism has
plagued the human mind for several thousand years and still
does so in different forms. Man has always felt that his actions
were free and that, therefore, he was responsible for his actions.
At the same time, he has had a strong sense that he is a victim
and tool of fortune, a Calvinistic God, his environment, or some
such force. Philosophers have tried to solve this dilemma in
many different ways and have succeeded as well as they could
with reason; that is, they have never really satisfied the human
mind because reason forces them to tilt the balance one way or
another. An Aquinas' elaborate facade of intermediary matters
does not disguise his bias towards predestination. On the other
hand, anyone who has watched *Oedipus Rex* on stage knows
and understands both sides of the problem without choosing one
over the other. The audience sees Oedipus acting freely at each
stage of the story and at the same time realizes that his every
free act brings him closer to fulfilling the destiny embodied in
the Delphic Oracle. Much of the controversy over this play turns
not upon any ambiguity in the story itself but on the confusion
of the critical mind, which can only express itself in rational
terms, when it wants to explain the myth. To take another example, the myth of the Fall makes one understand a fundamental problem in a way reason cannot. Man has always believed
that he and his world are basically good and yet that he is the
cause of evil in this world. In the Genesis myth the auditor sees
God make the world and man and call them good and then sees
man commit evil. He may not be able to explain rationally why
man acted as he did—Augustine did not succeed in solving the
problem of evil—but he understands, though in a different
thought-mode. The Renaissance critics invariably contended, and
I think rightly, that myth and allegory require a different response
altogether from that demanded by discursive reason and can be

applied to basic human problems just as reason can and, perhaps, with more success (to add my own opinion). The secrets behind the veil were mythic answers to the ultimate questions: What is man? How is he related to his surroundings? What is love? What is death? Despite this recognition, Renaissance critics could not avoid, any more than we can, trying to explain myth; and allegorical interpretation represents this inevitable conversion of myth into reason. In this attempt they also could not avoid using the rational categories of their own time, any more than a modern student of myth can. Frazer's agricultural explanations of myth are a variation on euhemerism, as Jung's archetypes represent a modern version of Pico's explanations in depth. What was unfortunate in the Renaissance was that serious myth was thrown out of literature, and the moral allegory which survived had no depth, deprived as it was of its basis in fundamental human problems. People had confused the rational interpretation of myth with its thought-form, for myth is open-ended. The complexity and rationalizations lie in its interpretations, and these will vary from one age to another, according to current ideas.

In this fact one can find a useful corrective for our own preconceptions about literature. We tend to equate profundity with complexity, but a myth is always profound and seldom complex. Or rather, complexity can be applied as a term to two different things: the work itself and the mind of the critic. A myth has a simple form but creates a complex response in its audience, while a novel may be complex both in form and in its understanding. A myth like that of Perseus and Medusa or that of the Fall could not be simpler in form, but it provokes complex responses on a profound level from its critics, and always will, because a myth is open-ended and demands completion on the part of an audience. Hence the numerous levels of allegory in the Renaissance or the many ironic and paradoxical readings of our own contemporaries. But all these interpretations indicate the difficulties of the critical mind, bound to rational discourse and trying to get at the profound suggestions inherent in myth. None of this variety should be allowed to veil the fact that the myth or the basic allegorical plot has a distressingly simple form. The Renaissance critics were absolutely correct when, in their attempt to explain the secrets of myth, they went behind the form of the myth into the mind of the poet, for in myth complexity lies in the mind and not in the form. At the same time this simplicity in myth might cause us to reconsider our high estimation of complexity. There are many complex works which are not profound at all. Donne can lead his auditors around an extraordinarily complicated argument or pseudoargument, but he may not have been profound in that argument. Similarly, a social novel, with its complex presentation of many characters, affecting and changing each other, may be superficial on fundamental questions. Applied to the form of a work, the two concepts may even be opposed—the more profundity, the less complexity. Milton justifies the ways of God to man as long as he sticks to the myth; but, when he has God justify his actions in rational terms, he fails. In those passages he alienates a modern audience and certainly does not convince them of his profundity. His story, on the other hand, still works because it is myth and can be reassessed in every succeeding age. One might say that myth and allegory are always simple, profound, and relevant—whatever the fashionable ideas of a period. They are of no age and for any age.

❧6❧

The Auditor's Response, Part Two

WE SAID EARLIER that the interpreter of allegory talked either about the broad outlines of the poet's myth or in detail about specific episodes or short poems. We must still discuss this latter operation. Henry Vaughan's well-known poem, *The Water-fall*, serves as a useful introduction to this kind of criticism because he made it into a dramatized exegesis of a particular symbol. The main concern of this chapter, however, will be with Spenser, and in particular with *The December Eclogue* of *The Shepheardes Calender* and with the *Hymn to Love*. What these analyses should demonstrate is the method of practical criticism and, more important, the kind of thinking allegory represents and the ends it serves. In some ways this criticism closely resembles modern approaches, but in others it is radically different.

I
The Water-fall

Henry Vaughan created in *The Water-fall* one of the few situations in which a modern can observe the process of allegorical criticism done by the author himself. The poem is reflexive, for the initial scene becomes the subject of the rest of the poem and goes through four interpretations: two psychological and two theological. Vaughan begins with a hieroglyph:

With what deep murmurs through times silent stealth
Doth thy transparent, cool and watry wealth
    Here flowing fall,
    And chide, and call,
As if his liquid, loose Retinue staid
Lingring, and were of this steep place afraid,
    The common pass
    Where, clear as glass,
    All must descend
    Not to an end:
But quickned by this deep and rocky grave,
Rise to a longer course more bright and brave.

The alternating pentameter and dimeter groups correspond to
the literal sense of the text: the lines become long when the poet
talks of the waters seeming to hang on the ledge above and
making a "longer course" below. They shorten and the quickly
recurring rhymes hurry the reader along when he refers to the
falling water itself. The scene contains or suggests its own interpretation. The water is men; the noise, their cries of fear and
resistance to death; the falling is the passage into death; the pool,
the grave, from which men arise to the longer life of eternity.

The hieroglyph in turn invites further explanation. As Plotinus remarks, such images appeal to the intuitive understanding,
but reason must explain them in a more extensive and discursive
fashion.[1] Vaughan goes on to rationalize this image of the falls,
changing the meter to a fixed tetrameter couplet as a sign. His
first analysis, perhaps inspired by the double falls, has two parts,
the one applied to the soul, the other to the body:

Dear stream! dear bank, where often I
Have sate, and pleas'd my pensive eye,
Why, since each drop of thy quick store
Runs thither, whence it flow'd before,
Should poor souls fear a shade or night,
Who came (sure) from a sea of light?

This exegesis depends upon a cosmological principle, what one

[1] *Enneads* 5. 8. 6.

might call the law of the conservation of water. Water falls to
the ground, sinks down and arises as a stream, flows to the
ocean, evaporates there and returns to its source as rain. Vaughan
applies this principle in a surprising fashion. Souls need not
fear shade or night, a statement which the reader ordinarily
would translate as sleep or death. But the sea of light implies a
different meaning. For the soul life on this earth is a death, a
lapse from the ever bright spheres of the sky into the darkness
of the sublunary world, a concept which Vaughan developed in
The World. The noisy fall then suggests the fear of souls to be
born.

The second analysis is less complex:

> Or since those drops are all sent back
> So sure to thee, that none doth lack,
> Why should frail flesh doubt any more
> That what God takes, hee'l not restore?

Here he shifts the emphasis, using the same principle as before.
No drop of water shall be lost. Similarly, the body should not
fear corruption and dissolution because it will be put back together again in the final resurrection. Already Vaughan has
changed the meaning of his hieroglyph three times, or rather,
discovered three different applications of the same symbol, depending on whether it was applied to men in general, to their
bodies, or to their souls.

His next two analyses are theological:

> O useful Element and clear!
> My sacred wash and cleanser here,
> My first consigner unto those
> Fountains of life, where the Lamb goes?

The water is Baptism, which enables the initiate to approach the
"fountains of life." Vaughan then explains what conditions make
an understanding of this symbolism possible:

> What sublime truths, and wholesome themes,
> Lodge in thy mystical, deep streams!

> Such as dull man can never finde
> Unless that Spirit lead his minde,
> Which first upon thy face did move,
> And hatch'd all with his quickning love.

The water is now associated with the primeval waters which covered chaos in the beginning of time, a common symbol in baptismal literature and one which widens the theological perspective to the limits of salvation history.[2] At the same time Vaughan has defined knowledge as life, for the Spirit which brought forth a world will illuminate the Christian and guide him to the "fountains of life." He is approaching a solution to the original problem suggested by the waterfall. He has shifted his emphasis and is now talking about a way to life and not about fear of death. In the final interpretation he passes to a positive longing for the next world:

> As this loud brooks incessant fall
> In streaming rings restagnates all,
> Which reach by course the bank, and then
> Are no more seen, just so pass men.

This idea enables him to reject the waterfall itself as an adequate object of contemplation and turn to the other fountains where the Lamb goes:

> O my invisible estate,
> My glorious liberty, still late!
> Thou art the Channel my soul seeks,
> Not this with Cataracts and Creeks.

Vaughan has resolved his problem, turning fear of death into a desire for eternal life. He can, therefore, reject his hieroglyph for one of the things that it suggested. The symbol gives way to a figural reality, the visible to the invisible.

    In the end the auditor realizes that Vaughan has charged his initial symbol with multiple levels of meaning, five to be

---

[2] See, for example, the Preface for the Blessing of the Font, which occurs on Easter Eve in the Roman Rite.

exact, some of them almost mutually contrary. To create these multiple meanings, he isolated each time a particular aspect of his symbol and used it as the basis for his interpretation, now the waterfall itself, now the drops of water, now the rings in the pool at the bottom. This technique was familiar to the old scriptural commentators, for Stephen Langton habitually employed it in his classroom lectures four hundred years earlier.[3]

What should strike a modern as most unusual in this technique is the mode of thought it manifests. No critic today would explicate Vaughan's hieroglyph in the manner in which Vaughan does because there is nothing in the text to warrant his interpretations. The only one supported by the text would be Vaughan's equation of the waterfall with the body's innate fear of decomposition. The others have no basis in the hieroglyph. A waterfall is not a symbol for baptism, as far as I know. One would expect a fountain or a well. To get at baptism a critic must think of the waterfall simply as water and ignore its specific form. Similarly, to think of the waterfall as souls fearing birth requires a critic to discount the explicit statements within the hieroglyph itself, which equate the falls with physical death and the grave. No modern critic could make this kind of interpretation because it violates the text. In other words, modern critical practice will not suffice for allegorical poetry. We are accustomed to look to the text for our understanding, but we must learn instead to think allegorically. We must enter into the poet's own mind and discover his mode of thought.

An example might help to explain this point more clearly. To make sense of the poem, one critic found it necessary to define the word *restagnates* according to its Latin meaning. Actually, he was solving a pseudoproblem because he ignored the allegorical mode of thought. Starting with the hieroglyph, he correctly identified the falls with death but then found Vaughan's last interpretation impossible to comprehend because

[3] Beryl Smalley, *The Study of the Bible in the Middle Ages* (Oxford, 1941), p. 198.

it contradicted his original meaning. Here is the passage and his comment:[4]

> As this loud brooks incessant fall
> In streaming rings restagnates all,
> Which reach by course the bank, and then
> Are no more seen, just so pass men.

. . . On the metaphorical level, with the waterfall representing death, the soul of man cannot possibly become stagnant again, since it is passing into heaven and no stagnation is possible there.

He expects Vaughan to maintain the same equations all the way through the poem. If the falls is death and the pool the grave at the beginning, then the pool cannot mean something else later on. So he constructs an improbable definition of *restagnates* as "to run over, overflow," and concludes absurdly:

> If the waterfall represents, as Francis asserts, death, then man, in imitating the waterfall, purifies himself at the point of death and through the act of dying. His soul bubbles up and overflows, casting off the impurities of life.

Such nonsense is not entirely due to the critic. He worships his texts like the rest of us and expects a set of meanings, once established, to be continued through the remainder of the poem. When he finds the train taking a wrong turning, he tries desperately to switch back to the original track. But the allegorist, unfortunately, does not think in his fashion and likes to go in several different directions, some of them quite unpredictable from the symbols and meanings with which he begins. As we shall see again in Spenser, an allegorist can find meanings in a text for which there is absolutely no verbal basis, and he may even reverse his original meanings. In effect, he makes of his original symbol whatever meaning he chooses; it has no fixed signification. For us this rather unsettling practice indicates that it is not enough to scan a Renaissance text with over-subtle eyes. We must learn to think allegorically, if we wish to cope success-

[4] Ted Larry Pebworth, "The Problem of *Restagnates* in Henry Vaughan's 'The Water-fall,' " *Papers on Language and Literature*, 3 (1967), 259.

fully with the poets of the period. We must bring back the *poeta* into our discussion of the *poema*.

II

Besides illustrating allegorical exegesis, *The Water-fall* likewise indicates the peculiar use of sense images in such poetry. Vaughan presents the hieroglyph of the falls in a strong sensual way, exploiting sound, line length, and rhyme in a combined appeal to the senses of hearing and sight. But in the course of the poem he takes his audience further and further away from this sense image, as he penetrates more and more into its allegorical meaning. Once he has achieved a theological understanding of the symbol, he discards it altogether, retaining only a figure for an invisible world of value, revealed to him by the Spirit. Much allegorical imagery functions in this manner. Sensual effects are heightened, and the image at first seems to exist as an end in itself, so forcefully is it presented. But the more the critic considers the image, the more he realizes that its function is almost antisensual. Sometimes, in fact, the image is so distorted that it defies visualization.

Spenser generally keeps his descriptions within the realm of vision, but they have a tendency to slide off from the symbol to the thing which it signifies. In most cases he conceals this shift amid a mass of concrete details and does not make it obvious, as Vaughan does for the waterfall. Take, for example, his description of Spring in the Mutabilitie Cantoes:

> So, forth issew'd the Seasons of the yeare;
>> First, lusty *Spring*, all dight in leaues of flowres
>> That freshly budded and new bloosmes did beare
>> (In which a thousand birds had built their bowres
>> That sweetly sung, to call forth Paramours):
>> And in his hand a iauelin he did beare,
>> And on his head (as fit for warlike stoures)
>> A guilt engrauen morion he did weare;
> That as some did him loue, so others did him feare.

$$[FQ\ 7.\ 7.\ 28]$$

At first glance this seems to be a very graphic picture, and the auditor can easily visualize someone dressed in leaves and flowers, carrying a javelin and wearing a gilt helmet. But one detail makes this simple picture grotesque and exaggerated. Who could imagine someone walking around with a thousand birds on his clothes? This distortion passes almost without notice because Spenser has just been talking about leaves and flowers, and birds in the trees seem a natural follow-up. Actually, he has gone beyond his symbol to the general fact of spring, where a thousand birds do build their nests and chirp love songs. For the attentive auditor such deliberate distortions would lead him behind the veil to the truth. This is a common technique with allegorical poets: to overwhelm the senses with a strong image and impress the memory and yet, at the same time, to distort the image and create a nonvisual effect. Spenser simply does it less obtrusively than others.

Spenser's distortions do become obvious and confusing to his audience when he places his images in an extended narrative. The dragon fight in Book One provides a celebrated example. Spenser makes his dragon of cosmic proportions, since it represents the Ancient Serpent which swept down a third of the stars in its fall (*FQ* 1. 11. Arg.). It is as large as a hill or mountain (11. 4, 8), its tail alone extends nearly 600 feet (11. 11) and can knock rocks into pieces and overthrow tall trees (11. 37). The dragon roars like a hundred lions (11. 37), and the blood from its wound would run a watermill (11. 22). But in the battle scenes the size of the dragon contracts. When it tries to fly off with horse and rider, it cannot carry them far enough. Like a hawk struggling to take off a "hardie fowle," it fails because the horse and rider are too heavy (11. 19). This is quite impossible if the dragon has the size Spenser gives him, for a six to seven hundred-foot monster could easily carry a knight and horse. Spenser covers up this discrepancy as well as he can by ignoring it. He describes the dragon in one way but tacitly assumes much smaller proportions during the actual battle. The attentive auditor again would perceive in this discrepancy a rent in the veil of allegory. Spenser must insist on the gigantic size of his dragon because he wants it to represent the apocalyptic dragon, but at the same time Saint George must kill his own mythic beast. Since no human being can really fight a cosmic dragon—they are generally left to angels and gods, to Saint Michael and Thor—he must contract the size of his serpent for the realistic details of his fight, while he expands its size for the symbolism.

This method of deliberate distortion should suggest a caveat on the many useful studies which have been made recently in iconography. For instance, Robert Kellogg and Oliver Steele in their edition of Spenser's first two books (1965) relate the dragon fight to a picture of Vittore Carpaccio. They draw many ingenious and illuminating points of comparison between the two, saying that "Carpaccio's fresco is detailed and very much in the spirit of Spenser's story."[5] But in one crucial particular Carpaccio is not at all in the spirit of Spenser. His dragon is of the small, domestic variety, about the size of Saint George's horse, not a mountain-like creature covering acres of landscape. Iconography serves as a useful guide only within certain limits because it does not really correspond to the techniques of allegorical poetry. The painter pours his meaning into his images, and his critics discover all they wish through his figures. In allegorical poetry, on the other hand, the critic must always be conscious of the poet's mind which controls these images. The poet may change them around at will, and the critic must watch the poet as well as his pictured veil.

Spenser provides the most notorious example of this image-shifting in his Garden of Adonis. As Thomas Roche remarks: "Problems arise when we try to visualize the place."[6] Concerned as he is more with the meaning of the Garden than with its

[5] Edmund Spenser, *Books I and II of* The Fairie Queene, ed. R. Kellogg and O. Steele (New York, 1965), p. 11.

[6] Thomas Roche, *The Kindly Flame* (Princeton, 1964), p. 120.

technique of imagery, Roche does not develop this comment
and dismisses the imagery earlier by saying, "Most of the detail in
this section lead the reader away from a precise visualization of
the scene toward the concepts that the garden represents."⁷ The
general purport of this statement is perfectly true and bears out
what I have been arguing, but Roche errs, I think, when he implies that the pictorial imagery is vague like that of Milton's
hell. Rather, it is quite precise, though contradictory, because
Spenser describes the Garden in three different ways, depending
upon the problem with which he is immediately concerned.
First of all, he presents the Garden as the seminary of all forms,
a place where forms grow like flowers. At the front gate Genius
clothes these forms in flesh and sends them out into the world.
They return eventually by the back door, once they have undergone fleshly corruption, and are then planted anew. This characterization of the forms suggests a generalization to Spenser:
forms die and change; matter or substance alone endures. With
this idea in mind Spenser shifts his description of the Garden
slightly and puts into it Time, who flies about cutting down the
forms in their separate plots. This description is perfectly clear
and well symbolizes the comment:

> The substance is not chaunged, nor altered,
> But th'only forme and outward fashion.
>   [3. 6. 38]

The fertile soil remains, though the plants may die. But if this
description is combined with the earlier one and read as a single
picture, everything becomes confused. In the first Time was
outside the Garden, now he is inside. This confusion compounds
itself because Spenser immediately modulates into yet another
description of the Garden, where it becomes a regular *locus
amoenus* with birds singing in the trees and boys and girls making
love in the grass. Spenser has shifted his symbols again because
he wishes to solve the problem of mutability through the figure

---

⁷ Ibid., p. 119.

of Adonis, who is both "Father of all formes" and "eterne in mutabilitie" (3. 6. 47). A critic who tries to reconcile these three descriptions can only fail. How can he explain forms or plants making love and flying around in the trees, or Time who is both in and not in the Garden? He can always accuse Spenser of confusion and say that the poet had a muddled mind, but he misses the point. Spenser is no more muddled here than is the writer of Revelation who goes over the destruction of the world several times through the imagery of the bowls, seals, and trumpets. The theme is the important thing—the truth behind the veil—, and the symbols may shift around or become distorted without warning, if truth requires it.

It is this image technique which most dismays a modern reader, trained as he is in symbolist criticism. English poetry since the Renaissance tends to make images fixed centers of meaning. Yeats' Byzantine artists created a golden tree which is sufficient unto itself and a point of immense significance to the poet. Or in *Tintern Abbey*, whatever the state of mind and feelings of Wordsworth, the landscape around the Abbey remains a fixed thing in his memory, a basis for reflection. This kind of imagery, whether symbolist or romantic, can be described by the old phrase: poetry is a speaking picture. The landscape may be external or within the mind, but it must be a landscape. Modern critics unconsciously apply this same principle when they try to explain allegorical poetry by contemporary pictures. When they find that the poetry responds only in a limited way to picture interpretations, they can always fall back on the old cliché that allegory is too abstract and does not allow its symbols full play. For example, no Renaissance artist, as far as I know, would paint three different pictures of the Garden of Adonis, changing its nature according to certain intellectual problems which he wishes to explain. He might create a narrative in three pictures but not this kind of superintellectual repetition. The allegorist seems to be too abstract and mental in his art. But this old accusation again misses the point. The allegorist is not talking in pictures but creating a mode of discourse. He does not serve his symbols; they serve him. He throws out various images and shifts them around, trying to get his auditors to participate in his own train of thought, which is both concrete and abstract. He does not meditate upon his symbols and separate the mental from the concrete; he uses his symbols for others, as guides to his meditation. To repeat an earlier principle, allegories are open-ended, and the critic tries to complete them and recover the same vision the poet once had. The *poema* depends upon the *poeta*.

It follows then that allegory should not be fitted into symbolist critiques or Aristotelian formulas. It demands, rather, what William Nelson calls "thematic criticism." The next two explanations—of *The December Eclogue* and *The Hymn to Love*—will provide examples of what I mean. At the same time they will be couched in the traditional terms of Renaissance criticism. I will talk in terms of "levels," that is, of different thematic questions.

III
The Hymn to Love

The main purpose of our discussion of *The Hymn to Love* will be to elucidate a general principle of allegorical criticism. It is the principle of which distorted imagery forms a part, and it provided the means by which the poet could force his audience to go from the lower to the higher levels of allegory. Lodge briefly enunciates this principle in his argument with Gosson. He quotes Campano, saying "The vanitie of tales is wonderful; yet if we aduisedly looke into them they wil seme and proue wise." Chapman refers to this absurdity principle in his Letter to Somerset, when he says of the *Odyssey:* "If the Bodie (being the letter, or historie) seemes fictiue, and beyond Possibilitie to bring into Act: the sence then and Allegorie (which is the soule) is to be sought."[8] Classical authorities show more fully how this principle operates. According to the Emperor Julian, the poet creates in his literal fiction certain absurdities which cannot be accounted for on the literal-moral levels of the allegory and so require a philosophical explanation. As he says, "Whenever myths or sacred subjects are incongruous in thought, by that very fact they cry aloud, as it were, and summon us not to believe them literally but to study and track down their hidden meaning. And in such myths the incongruous element is even more valuable than the serious and straightforward. . . ."[9] More valuable because the absurd exposes the fiction as fiction and does not allow an audience to rest content with it.[10] The distortions of allegorical imagery, which we discussed earlier, fulfill precisely this function. They draw attention away from an illusionary, surface realism to an inward truth. They form one part of the absurdist principle. Origen, who applies this principle to sacred Scripture, explains its rhetorical function in more detail. A coherent literal myth might completely satisfy an audience and thus foil the speaker's purpose.[11] The artist wants to convey a message to his audience, not to entertain them. Or, rather, he wants to entertain them only to the extent that they become curious about the meaning behind his stories. Therefore, somewhere or other, he must discredit his fiction to win credence for his point of view. The story must remain incomplete or absurd, if the poet wants to let truth shine through his pictured veil.

Spenser may have been using this principle when he cut out of *The Faerie Queene* the reunion of Scudamour and Amoret. Their literal story is not his main concern, and this violation of the narrative may have been his method of turning his auditors

[8] For Lodge, see Smith, 1: 65; for Chapman, see the *Poems of George Chapman*, ed. Phyllis Bartlett (New York, 1962), p. 407.

[9] *Oration* 7. 117.

[10] *Oration* 5. 475.

[11] *Peri.* 4. 2. 9. Rufinus' version draws more attention to the problems of narrative.

away from a surface understanding of his allegory. In this particular case we can never be certain, for the omission may have been caused by hasty rearrangement before the publication of the Second Part of *The Faerie Queene.* But in *The Hymn to Love* his use of this absurdity principle is quite clear and unquestioned.

To begin with the literal level. Spenser presupposes the world of classical myth. The poet promises to raise Love "Boue all the gods" (304), if his prayers are answered, and he has Hercules and Hebe inhabit a classical heaven. Love has conquered the speaker of the poem and has inflicted on him considerable suffering. For relief the speaker will honor Love in song by a story of his triumphs, hoping thereby to gain favor from his tormentor. He follows the conventions of such poems[12] and includes a full genealogy of the god and a history of his notable deeds, ending with a request, which this speaker skillfully presents as the end of his story, in which Love opens to the noble lover a paradise of pleasure. He too like Hercules would ascend Olympus and marry Hebe. This request remains unanswered, and, like the Chaucer of the *Parlement,* the narrator closes his poem with a sense of his own exclusion from the joys which he has described. Nevertheless, the dominant tone of the hymn is positive.

The rhetorical function of this fiction differs markedly from what we shall see in the *Calender.* Spenser has an established reputation as a poet and can speak in his own person, as he does in *The Faerie Queene.* He chooses the form of the hymn, which Puttenham considers to be the highest type of poetry, including drama and epic. His stanza is the rhyme royal, a recognized vehicle for serious poetry.[13] The humility which colors the poem is that of the poet addressing his divinities and the lover supplicating his mistress, but to his audience Spenser need make no apologies. The fiction likewise has a private and practical end, which Spenser states explicitly in the next hymn. He prays to

---

[12] Puttenham, *Arte* 1. 12.
[13] Gascoigne, *Certayne Notes of Instruction,* 14. In Smith, 1: 54.

Love to win his mistress. Thus, the poem presents two aspects: a description of the love process and an attempt to realize that process in his own life. The whole handling of the myth is dynamic and positive.

The history naturally contains its own moral, stressed by the one defective stanza of the *Hymn*. Nelson has already discussed this matter sufficiently, so a brief summary will serve our purpose.[14] Noble lovers, in the same situation as the speaker of the poem, break out of their bonds by action and translate sentiment into chivalric heroism. The blind Cupid symbolizes this process and explains it:

> Thou art his god, thou art his mightie guyde,
> Thou being blind, letst him not see his feares,
> But cariest him to that which he hath eyde,
> Through seas, through flames, through thousand swords and
>   spears:
> Ne ought so strong that may his force withstand,
> With which thou armest his resistlesse hand.
>
>   [225-30]

Success rewards the lover's virtuous deeds, and he finds "grace" with his lady. The baseborn lover cannot endure this initial situation, for he falls in love at first sight and expects an immediate reciprocation of his advances. Time then separates the baseborn and noble lovers. The former cannot wait nor will he turn love into heroic action. The moral here is not unexpectedly a cliché, not only of medieval romance but of classical literature as well. In the *Symposium* Plato expresses the same idea through the character of Pausanias.

On this level, however, the poem does not make adequate sense. Spenser has strewn his tale with absurdities and paradoxes, none of which can be resolved by a moral analysis. The speaker's rhetorical situation provides the first example of this calculated "vanitie." In this hymn the speaker seems to have fallen into a strange psychological state which ironically qualifies the high

---

[14] Nelson, p. 101.

moral claims of the narrative. Tormented by love, the speaker tries to escape from his situation by flattery—of his tormentor. One obstacle might prevent him from completing his moral surrender: his wits have been enfeebled by all the suffering which he has endured. He can only hope that Love himself will aid him in his task, rather an odd hope, since Love put him in this situation in the first place. The speaker is in a psychological and moral cul-de-sac. Love has ruined him, and yet only Love can save him.

The *Hymn* becomes stranger as it goes along. The speaker thinks that Love has *three* parents: Venus, Plenty, and Penury. He is elder than his birth and a perennial child, though older than all the gods. Worse, the narrator interrupts his story in one place to ask some embarrassing questions. Why should he honor someone who grants him no favors? Why does Love punish his own subjects, especially since history shows that he is the "worlds great Parent" (156)? The answer given, though conventional, seems initially unsatisfactory. Love torments his subjects to make them better deserve a reward and to make the reward more esteemed.

A successive cosmological-psychic allegory explains this answer. Again, since Nelson has discussed this level extensively, we need only summarize the theme.[15] In the Orphic myth, Love, awakened by Necessity (Clotho) and enlightened by his mother Venus, creates the cosmos and maintains it in existence by generation. In all creatures he has infused a fire which drives them to reproduce themselves, but "man, that breathes a more immortall mynd,/Not for lusts sake, but for eternitie,/ Seekes to enlarge his lasting progenie" (103-5). The suffering lover is really fulfilling man's unique end, established by Love at the beginning of time. His psychological crisis is part of an established cosmic pattern. His torments, both before and after his lady grants him "grace," signify his progressive disengagement from "all sordid basenesse" (191) and the remolding of his mind "Vnto a fairer forme" (193) which excells his own thought. His chivalric accom-

15 Ibid., pp. 100-101.

plishments visibly manifest this reformation and win him "grace," but he still must pass through the purgatory of jealousy before he escapes the world into an innocent paradise of love. Pleasure is his "lasting progenie," or his specifically human participation in the maintenance of the cosmos. She is the daughter of Cupid and Psyche, of Love acting in the Mind and controlling the body (43-44). Thus, the psychic allegory depends upon the prior cosmological allegory for its own meaning. The principle of generation explains the lover's plight.

The psychic allegory also relates to the first dialectically. The individual lover, rising above himself, imitates the cosmic flight of Eros, and they both in a sense create worlds: the one, the world of time, the other, an eternal world of pleasure. They both have double parents: the beauty which awakens love in the individual is Venus, the Queen of Beauty and the pattern by which Eros made the world, while the Tantalus-like lover, ever longing for more in the midst of plenty, explains the parentage of Plenty and Penuria.[16] The two levels also explain the confusing statement that Eros is older than his birth and a perennial child, though older than the gods. Love is constantly being born on the human level, though as a cosmic principle he existed before the world was made. But all this resemblance between the cosmological and psychological levels aggravates some important differences. The two levels also oppose each other as beginning and end. Love makes the world of time, but the lover escapes from it into an eternal world of pleasure: the individual human being reverses the pattern of creation. But, "Like as two mirrours by opposd reflexion" (*Hymn to Beauty* 181), the two allegories really express the same mystery, viewed in different perspectives, that of the cosmos and that of the individual. The poem turns in upon itself, for one part refers to and depends upon the other.

This philosophical allegory dominates the poem and explains away the absurdities embedded in the literal narrative. It is the end to which the euhemeristic myth leads, the truth behind the

[16] See *Amoretti* 83 for an exact analogue.

veil. And yet there is a further truth behind the philosophical truth, for the hymn contains a theological dimension. This level contrasts sharply with the determined classicism of the literal level and at the same time is necessary for the poet's rhetorical situation. What can one say of a poet who addresses a Christian audience and yet pretends to live solely in the world of classical myth, which can only appear as vanity to his auditors? His very choice demands some kind of theological explanation. Spenser insures a theological level for his hymn by adding the Heavenly Hymns, which both present a Christian viewpoint in themselves and point to the hidden theology of *The Hymn to Love*, something a modern critic might well miss. Nothing in the text itself justifies this kind of interpretation.

As Nelson has shown, Spenser creates a house of mirrors out of his *Fowr Hymnes*, for the poems all have the same arrangement and the same general topic.[17] So *The Hymn to Love* resembles *The Hymn to Beauty* as effect to cause; it resembles *The Hymn to Heavenly Love* in a common subject matter; and the first two hymns resemble the last two as earthly shadows to heavenly realities. These juxtapositions of themselves create a new understanding of *The Hymn to Love*, for the presence of two things similar but not the same makes metaphor and allegory possible, and in the perspective of *The Heavenly Hymns* *The Hymn to Love* can be interpreted as theological allegory, translating its original meaning "to another not proper, but yet nigh and like."[18] *The Hymn to Beauty*, while it complements the ideas in the first hymn, does not add another level to the auditor's understanding.

Spenser arranged his *Heavenly Hymns* in the manner of Ficino's commentary on Plato's *Symposium*. Ficino made his *Banquet* resemble the original in form as well as in subject matter, so that he mirrored one art work with another, which itself depended upon the original for a full understanding and at the

---

17 Nelson, pp. 99 ff.
18 Peacham, *Garden*, p. 3.

same time enriched that original with all the ideas and subtleties of the later Platonic tradition. The two works mutually qualify each other and are to be read together. Spenser likewise designed his *Heavenly Hymns* as theological correctives to his original hymns, for he wanted to remedy the abuses which the young made out of their misunderstanding of the two earthly hymns.[19] The two later hymns, therefore, provide a commentary to the earlier hymns and presuppose the existence of these hymns in their own construction.

Similarly, *The Hymn to Heavenly Love* makes possible a Christian understanding of the Eros myth and the paradise of pleasure described in *The Hymn to Love*. Thomas Roche suggests this idea in passing when he says that the parallelism of the Four Hymns invites theological allegory, but he does not argue that the earthly hymn itself fits a Christian theological pattern.[20] Nor does Nelson, who elaborates the various points of comparison between the two hymns. Actually, Spenser made of his classical hymn the kind of theological allegory which we have already seen in Boccaccio's *Pantheon* or in Golding's version of Ovid. Golding had argued that the *order* of Ovid's narrative corresponded to the order of events in Genesis, and Spenser has arranged his classical history in a similar fashion. Spenser's Love first needs light, then he separates the four elements into pure and mixed, keeping them within certain limits, and finally commands that all creatures propagate themselves. God on the first day created light, and on the second, according to Pico's version of Genesis (*Hep.* 1. 3), he separated the elements into pure and mixed and established their limits, a process which the biblical narrator symbolized by the creation of the firmament and the separation of the land from the sea. Having made the creatures of the world, God commanded them: "Be fruitful, and multiply." This command Spenser images in prophetic terms as

[19] See his Dedicatory Letter to the Countesses of Cumberland and Warwick.

[20] Roche, pp. 124-25.

a fire burning within the creature.[21] The recreating of the human being through love symbolizes in profane terms the mystery of salvation, while the voluptuous paradise of pleasure, seemingly so epicurean and unplatonic, images the restored Eden. Reynolds interprets the word *Eden* conventionally as the Greek *ēdonē* and Latin *voluptas* and explains that the Garden of Eden was a garden of delight without sin, actually before sin existed.[22] Spenser twice emphasizes the sinless character of the lovers' pleasures:

> There with thy daughter *Pleasure* they doe play
> Their hurtlesse sports, without rebuke or blame,
> And in her snowy bosome boldly lay
> Their quiet heads, deuoyd of guilty shame.
>
> [287-90]

But again Spenser has reversed the Creation pattern. His lovers enjoy pleasure after sin, not before, for they have passed through purgatory into "heauens glorie" (279). The earthly hymn in all its relevant details foreshadows a heavenly reality.

After reading this analysis of *The Hymn to Love*, one might well be surprised how close this kind of criticism comes to modern methods. Before this chapter we have emphasized the unicity of allegorical rhetoric and its essential differences from other modes of persuasion. In the previous chapter the discussion of the levels made allegory even stranger. No one today would approach a myth in the manner of Boccaccio and Pico. But, when it comes to the criticism of actual texts, the modern exegete can find most of the levels on his own. Nelson moves freely from moral to philosophical levels, and for this reason I used his interpretation as much as possible. He demonstrates how close modern criticism has come to allegorical criticism. This similarity, however, masks some important differences. We gen-

---

[21] *HL* 92-105. For a prophetic analogue, see Jer. 5:14.
[22] In Spingarn, 1: 176. The idea is at least as old as Clement of Alexandria. See *Strom.* 2.11.

erally do not connect the levels, ladder-fashion, nor do we assume that absurdities in the narrative function as stairways leading to the other levels. We are so trained in symbolist criticism that improbabilities on the literal level often do not register. When Spenser assigns three parents to Love, the Platonic reference lights up in the critic's mind, and he goes on reading without any difficulty. In fact, he reads habitually on several levels at once. It takes a flagrant abuse of the literal narrative to awake a modern critic, like Spenser's "confused" description of the Garden of Adonis or his omission of the reunion between Scudamour and Amoret. The allegorical critic, despite what may seem to us many wild notions, has a more controlled method of approaching a text. He asks one kind of question at a time and begins with the literal. The text will generally force him to change his level of questions, and then there will be no difficulties with the Garden of Adonis. Much more serious problems arise for the modern critic, however, in those instances where the text itself gives no obvious clues whatsoever. We could never do what Vaughan did to his hieroglyph or what I just did to *The Hymn to Love*. The text must warrant the interpretation, and these theological levels simply are not in it. Spenser never mentions Christ in his *Hymn*, but his Eros does in fact signify the Logos. But, if we are conscious of how the poet distorts his imagery and his narrative and know something of contemporary criticism, we will have learned to think like the poet and can interpret a text correctly even without obvious pointers given by the poet. Once we have learned to think thematically and concretely, always regarding symbols as means, not ends, most of the difficulties in allegory should disappear. And it is in these cases that the discipline of allegorical criticism becomes absolutely necessary. Allegorical poetry encourages wild commentary, as Fowler's book indicates, for the critic is voyaging upon strange seas of thought. He needs all the controls and precautions he can get if he wishes to find anything of value on his journey.

IV
The   December Aeglogue

Now that we have established a method of criticizing allegory, we must ask how the poet effects his purpose through the allegory and what that purpose is. My discussion of the *Shepheardes Calender* and the *December Eclogue* in particular will be directed toward this end. Again, as in the preceding analysis, I will deliberately draw into my discussion representative modern critics, to show that we have in fact done much of this already. It is easy for a student, confronted with the *Heptaplus*, to conclude that Renaissance and modern critical methods have little in common. Actually they have much in common, and a study like this would have been impossible without the developments in criticism since 1940.

On the literal level Nelson has shown that Spenser deliberately chooses a negative euhemeristic myth for two related purposes.[23] In one respect Spenser, as a beginning poet, must mask himself in humble weeds, for he has to approach his audience with proper humility, apologizing for his lack of skill and promising little. He dons the disguise of a "Shepheards boye (no better doe him call)" (*Jan.* 1). At the same time he tries to build up his own ethos and convince his audience of his real abilities. The rustic Colin enjoys certain advantages in his world which the poet Spenser does not have in his own, namely the recognition from his peers which the fledgling poet has still to win. Further, *December* assigns to Colin almost mythic status. His woes come to him from a god, angered at the shepherd's hubris, who competed with the divine. But Spenser keeps this praise within due bounds. He has Colin admit in *December* how rude his songs appear when compared to those of Pan and, implicitly, how ridiculous a shepherd's hubris can be. On the other hand, this disclaimer, true though it is to the world of the poem, rings false for the poet Spenser, and is intended to. The dazzling variety of verse pat-

23 Nelson, pp. 30-32.

terns and in particular the sophisticated forms ascribed to Colin Clout belie the humility. One might characterize Spenser's fiction as negative euhemerism with constant suggestions of the opposite.

This negative pattern continues on the moral level of the allegory. Spenser wishes to warn his audience away from love. Both a modern like Nelson and an Elizabethan like E. K. make this point. Nelson talks of "the theme of love the destroyer," and *December* sums up this moral for the *Calender*. Love has destroyed Colin's career as a poet:[24]

> The rage of love, kindled in the young man's breast by the god of shepherds ("But better mought they have behote him Hate"), blasts the promised harvest. On this dark note the *Calender* ends.

E. K. ascribes two moral ends to the *Calender*, but they are really the same as Nelson's single end. First, he says that Spenser wrote his eclogues for cathartic purposes. Caught in the throes of an unhappy love, he tried to mitigate the heat of his passion by singing about it. To complain of love is to purge it, according to the old medical principle: *similia similibus curantur*. Second, E. K. presents Spenser's own explanation, which is that he wants to warn other people away from the follies of love. But these two purposes are really the same because to complain of love is to warn others away from it: both present the theme of love the destroyer.

As on the literal level, a positive side to this moral polemic does appear now and then. Thenot praises Colin's songs to Rosalind (*Nov.* 43-44), and Piers' belief is not wholly discounted— that love can raise man out of the dust. And there is the familiar cliché that Colin's renunciations of poetry and life are themselves good poetry, filled with careful details drawn from rustic experience. The attitude is not totally negative; some light does gleam in the darkness, little though it may be.

[24] Ibid., p. 41.

On the philosophical level Spenser's departures from his normal method show his general purpose. Ordinarily, he follows the Florentine technique; that is, the characters of the *Calender* are defined by the cosmos. This works very well in the primitive conditions of the shepherd's life, for the rustic lives by the seasons. He rejoices in spring and sorrows in winter. So Colin refuses to sing a joyous song in *November* because it does not befit the time of the year, and Willy and Palinode think one should make merry in the spring.[25] The season determines the emotional states of the characters, but it can appear in other ways too. Thomalin in *July* makes the weather part of a psychological and moral argument. The heat should drive goatherds away from the exposed hill tops, just as the humble Christian should avoid the heights of ambition. Colin, more egocentrically, tends to see the landscape the other way around, as a mirror of his internal condition. So in the *August* sestina he chooses the wild woods in his lovelorn despair, and in *December* he defines what he sees in nature according to his psychological state. Before he fell in love, he found in the external world a positive state with bees and chanting birds, but afterward toadstools and ghastly owls came in their place. In all these passages he depends utterly on nature for the words he needs for introspection. The cosmos provides him with the terminology necessary for him to understand himself: his talents become flowers which Rosalind spilled or fruits rotted on the ground (103-14), and his girl a comet burning in the House of Venus (55-60). Thus, the characters mirror the landscape and sometimes the landscape mirrors the characters. As Hallett Smith remarks:[26]

> What does this leave for the spectator as a point of view? It is impossible to keep the position of the shepherd, for he is sometimes only a reflection of nature; it is impossible to keep the point of view of nature, for it is often only a reflection of the moods and feelings of the shepherd.

[25] *March* 1-6, *May* 1-16. Hallett Smith makes similar observations in his *Elizabethan Poetry* (Cambridge, Mass., 1964), p. 35.

[26] *Elizabethan Poetry*, p. 35.

On the rare occasions when a character opposes his reactions to the cosmos, Spenser reveals his attitudes and purpose. The joyous seasons are undercut. The glorious song of *April* is a song of the past, and major figures like Piers and Colin refrain from the spring merrymaking. Nelson has shown that Colin, though he can recognize the renewed Paradise which his friend Hobbinoll experiences on the "grassye ground with daintye Daysies dight" (June 6), cannot partake in that happy condition himself.[27] He lives without a refuge and cannot escape from a cruel fate. Rejoicing and fun are curiously absent from the *Calender*; the dominant note is one of lamentation. No one can escape from fate. The symbolism appears to be largely negative, something which Spenser arranged by his order of the months, which signifies this all-embracing fate. As E. K. admits, the poet could have begun the *Calender* in March, and this arrangement would have suggested a positive attitude, for it begins with spring and ends with winter's dying. Instead he chose January as his starting point, so that he could begin and end the *Calender* in dead winter. The seasons make a great circle, leading back to where they began with Colin shivering in the cold and lamenting his life. Colin is right for the world of this poem: man cannot escape a cruel fate with its seasons and signs of the zodiac, moving in a closed circle.

Spenser's treatment of human misery differs markedly here from its presentation in the Mutabilitie Cantoes. There man's circle of life became the means of human perfection. He could never achieve at any time the totality of human virtues but followed them through successively, as he passed from one stage of life to another. To paraphrase Nature's judgment, man dilates his being and achieves perfection through fate rather than in opposition to it. The strength and energy of youth give way to the judgment of middle age, and each period has its peculiar virtues. In this manner Nature confounds Mutabilitie and salves the ills which man had inherited from Adam. Neoplatonically, the pattern of the circle represented man's imitation of the eternal and

[27] Nelson, p. 49.

stable. But in the *Calender* the negative side of this circle is stressed, and all the evils of each season are noted and remembered. The circle of time and the seasons of the cosmos shut man up in a prison, from which he cannot break out. Here, as on the other levels, some positive attitudes are occasionally expressed. Hobbinoll did find a kind of Paradise in *June*, and the poetic rapture which Cuddie describes in *October* offers another kind of escape. But in both places these gleams of light disappear almost immediately. Colin cannot share in Hobbinoll's condition, and Hobbinoll's fate ironically depends upon that of his friend. In *October* Cuddie admits ruefully that poetic enthusiasms are not possible in his decadent society. Death offers the only real means of escape. Colin awaits it in *December*, though he sees it negatively, but in *November* he had characterized it as a door to a Paradise, where all the positive elements in his world remained and the negative ones were eliminated. By death alone can man break out of fate's charmed circle. On the other hand, as Smith has shown, this situation does not exist for the poet Spenser.[28] He appends to E. K.'s footnotes a little poem at the end of the *Calender*, and this afterword provides a very different answer to the circle. His *Calender* as an art work conquers time and mutation, for it will endure, always the same, until "the worlds dissolution" (4). His very representation of human futility conquers it and liberates man from the circle. The poet himself may succumb to time, but his work endures forever.

Any discussion of the purpose of allegory must eventually account for the different purposes of the different levels considered together. And here what strikes one as singular about the *Calender* is its uniform negative tone. This uniformity by no means comes of necessity. Theocritus, in his *Seventh Idyll*, combined a negative euhemerism with a positive over-view, and one can cite countless other examples. While in one respect a negative literal myth always involves a certain negative attitude toward individuals, it does not demand a negative philosophical

28 *Elizabethan Poetry*, pp. 40-41.

perspective. Spenser could debase himself as Colin Clout for rhetorical purposes, but he need not have inveighed against love or developed a *contemptus mundi* theme. Rather, the philosophical level provides the key to the negativism of the *Calender*. If a poet wishes to convince his audience of the futility of life, he will naturally turn his subject matter into an image and symbol of this attitude. So in the *Calender* love appears as a major catastrophe, a perfect emblem of cruel fate. It follows then, as we argued in the last chapter, that the inner core of allegory defines its principal purpose as rhetoric. The poet's inner truth or vision determines his end, not his figurative vehicle.

It remains for us to see what practical ends this negative rhetoric serves in Spenser's audience. Or, in other words, what would his auditors remember from the *Calender* and in particular from *December*, which sums it up? The average audience would carry away within them a strong sense of human futility and recall the image of the old poet, freezing in the cold and giving up. In this sense, the *Calender* creates a strong negative suasion in an auditor, a *contemptus mundi* mentality, heightened by the careful descriptions of the beauties of nature, which nevertheless are insufficient to alleviate man's condition in the cosmos. The only alternative to this situation is death, escape from the circle of time and change. But the elite audience will have experienced something quite different during the recitation of *December* and will recall this peculiar experience as much as the poem itself. They have viewed Colin Clout from a divine perspective, from which they can understand his problems with that combination of sympathy and detachment with which the Olympian gods watched the drama of Troy. That is, Spenser has captured time *within* the poem and placed his audience *outside* it. This experience itself, this standing outside the circle of time, answers the dilemmas of Colin Clout and, implicitly, of mankind. If man can escape from the circle, even for a moment, he must have within him something which transcends his environment. The poet through his art creates the conditions in which man can realize his Olympian qualities and by which he can gain the detachment necessary to live inside the circle. He may grow old and suffer, but he knows that he himself has broken out of this prison and can do so again.

This experience finds rational expression in the doctrine of poetic inspiration, an idea to which we have referred again and again. E. K. in his Argument for *October* credits Spenser with the theory that poetry is "no arte, but a diuine gift and heauenly instinct not to bee gotten by laboure and learning, but adorned with both: and poured into the witte by a certain *enthousiasmós*, and celestiall inspiration." Poetry comes to man from outside the circle, and those who participate in the poetic act automatically step into the "Ewiger Klarheit" of the gods.[29] The poet's allegories create for his auditors a pattern of responses and attitudes which, if they become habitual, forever remove them from the absolute control of mutability. One can say, therefore, that allegory or mythology finds its practical end in a mode of thought which itself liberates man from his environment and reveals to him his own transcendence.

In the *Calender* Spenser demonstrates the power of mutability through the content of his allegory, while the experience of his allegory provides a positive focus. The more he emphasizes the negative side of the human condition, the more necessary poetry becomes. It originates in divine inspiration, in superhuman vision, and has as its end the same experience for other people. So we return to the original point of this book. Without divine truth, allegory has no meaning as a rhetorical mode. And it is here that modern criticism fails. No one today can believe with Pico della Mirandola that Homer saw the ghost of Achilles in a vision and wrote the *Iliad* as a consequence.[30] We recognize the theory of divine inspiration as a historical fact, but we relegate it to a subordinate position, somewhere outside our real concerns. As a result we miss the principal purpose of allegory, which stems

---

[29] The phrase is from Hölderlin's *Hyperions Schicksalslied* 15.
[30] Reynolds quotes this passage. In Spingarn, 1: 151.

from this divine vision. The afflatus exists at the center of allegorical theory, not at its periphery.

Perhaps we have so much trouble in this respect because we still think of poetry as an end in itself rather than as a medium. The purpose of allegorical rhetoric is to create a particular experience within a person. The words of the poet stimulate this experience. Partial as it is, the *lógos prophorikós* requires the auditor to complete the poem himself, and in the process he enters into the thought-modes of the poet. He sees through the poet's verbal veil into the poet's mind and there finds truth, but a truth which does not correspond to our notions of truth. He finds not a fact or a concept but a way of looking at things which reveals to him his own divinity. As if he saw lightning flash in a clear night sky, he suddenly perceives that he, simply by being man, transcends his own world, and the more he thinks mythologically, the less he is bound by the chains of contingency. In Eliot's terms he stands "At the still point of the turning world" (*Burnt Norton* 2. 16), or as Rilke might say, he thinks angelically, seeing life and death as different aspects of the same whole.[31] Whatever critical or philosophical vocabulary we use to describe this experience, it does exist and it alone justifies the veil of allegory. The truth behind the painted veil is man himself.

Additional Remarks

For Spenser one might hazard a comment or two in regard to his theory of love and his Platonism, though two poems can hardly provide evidence for more than tentative statements. First of all, his attitudes to love. In the *December Eclogue* and *The Hymn to Love*, as well as in much of his other poetry, Spenser treats the problems of Eros. What one sees in the juxtaposition of these two poems is a shift from a negative to a positive attitude, a shift corroborated by *The Faerie Queene*, where the two

[31] See the Letter to his Polish Translator, which is quoted in the Leishman-Spender *Duino Elegies*, p. 93.

lovers, Britomart and Artegall, are successful in their love affair. At the same time, the elements of the problem do not change. In particular, the futility of the lover's situation plagued Spenser all his life, as it did most "courtly" love poets. Britomart symbolizes this futility most spectacularly, for she wanders off into strange lands, seeking a lover whom she has never met. This problem was given classic formulation two thousand years earlier by Aristophanes in his famous *Symposium* speech. The lover goes about the world looking for his other half; and, even if he is lucky enough to find his beloved, he still cannot attain a real unity with that person. Man is a part sundered from a whole which he can never regain.

Much of the strength of Petrarchan and courtly love poetry comes from its implicit recognition of this futility which bedevils any love affair. Despite all his idealism the Petrarchan is basically a realist because he begins more or less where other love poets like Catullus end—he realizes that the lover will never find adequate satisfaction. In a sense the Petrarchan has gone beyond the tragic, since he already knows the worst, or finds it out rather soon. But this knowledge is also his weakness as a poet, for where does one go from futility? The obvious answer is a simple renunciation of Eros, like that of Colin in the *December Eclogue*. His comments do not differ so much from the famous conclusion of Ronsard to his *Sonnets pour Helene*: "Car l'Amour & la Mort n'est qu'une mesme chose." But this variation on the *contemptus mundi* theme does not resolve anything: the lover simply washes his hands of the whole affair. It is to Spenser's credit that in *The Faerie Queene* and in the Platonic Hymns he moved beyond this negativism into a real solution. He took from Plato the idea that the lover's dissatisfaction indicates his essential humanity. Animals are content with brief pleasures and accept the *saeculum* in which they exist, but not men. Thus, Spenser's lover through his trials actually grows up and becomes heroic: he resists his situation and makes of himself a truly human person. He wrests his own salvation out of his futile condition. And his reward is Eden, something which Spenser did not find in Plato. The smiles, conversation, and kisses of his mistress recover for him the Paradise he lost through Adam. Despair need not lead to renunciation; it might open doors to rooms which man knew of only in dreams.

In a profound way Spenser's resolution of Eros mirrors his allegorical mode. In both the human being steps outside the circle of Fate and transcends his situation. Man can be liberated either by the Muses or by Eros. Thus, when Spenser chose love for his *Hymn*, he constructed a content which stated analogically the purposes of the form in which he wrote. Form and content relate to each other metaphorically and bear out Socrates' old contention—that love and poetry are two varieties of the same divine madness.[32] Poetic art cannot be developed much further than this.

One last comment. Nelson observes that Spenser's system of love, when examined logically, "disintegrates at once into a con-glomeration of inconsistencies and even absurdities."[33] This statement cannot be denied but probably could apply equally well to other mythological perspectives, whenever they suffer transformation into the language of reason. But they cannot be judged by their philosophical analogues, for they exist in their own right as a different mode of thought. And if we consider their very human function in society, we must take them seriously. Milton preferred Spenser to Aquinas. It follows that Spenser's shift from a negative to a positive attitude has real importance for the critic. Spenser began his career by contrasting unfavorably the mundane world and his divinely inspired vision. He later reconciled the two. The light which gleamed fitfully in the dark world of the *Calender* eventually illuminated the world. That he could go beyond contempt should have encouraged others, for the poet was their guide, the Hermes who led them into vision. His pattern could be theirs.

These two poems likewise shed light on the vexed question of the Florentine influence on Spenser's poetry, so ably restated

[32] *Phaedrus* 245.
[33] Nelson, p. 115.

by Robert Ellrodt in his *Neoplatonism in the Poetry of Spenser* (1960). While I do not quarrel with Ellrodt's specific points, it seems to me that his arguments lose their relevance in the wider context of allegory. All his life Spenser wrote the kind of allegory which the Florentines had revived, whether he had actually read them or not. The giveaway here is Spenser's constant stress on the cosmological level. The cosmos plays a major role in his early and in his later poetry, in *The Shepheardes Calender*, the *Hymns*, and *The Faerie Queene* with its Garden of Adonis and the Mutabilitie Cantoes. Not everyone in Tudor England shared with Spenser this fascination with the cosmos. Hawes did not, nor did Turbervile, Gascoigne, Sidney, and many other of Spenser's contemporaries and near contemporaries. He might not have found cosmic allegory in the classical dictionaries or even in Boccaccio, who does not so allegorize the Gorgon myth. But he could have found this stress in Golding or in the Florentines or perhaps in Alanus de Insulis and the other medieval predecessors of Pico and Ficino. His contemporary, Harington, had it, and so did Reynolds later. Whatever the mode of influence, these writers shared a common attitude toward allegory, and the cosmos determined much of their thought. They were classicists in the Renaissance sense of that term, disciples of men like the Emperor Julian and the Neoplatonists of the later Empire.

Spenser could not have known, of course, that this tradition was approaching extinction; in fact, today it is no longer recognized as classical. Reynolds in the next century was already a true John the Baptist, a voice crying in the wilderness. A revolution was taking place in Spenser's own time, for Gascoigne, Sidney, Puttenham, and the Ramists no longer identified poetry with allegory. By the time of Ben Jonson a new classicism had emerged, based upon the writers of the early Empire and parent to English neoclassicism. Allegory as a dominant form had disappeared, not to be revived till the end of the eighteenth century.

7

The End of Allegory

THE PUBLICATION of *The Faerie Queene* marked a kind of apogee in the history of allegorical rhetoric, a height not reached since Dante wrote *The Divine Comedy* three hundred years earlier. It also marked the end of the allegorical tradition. Even while Spenser was writing his great epic, his contemporaries were busy destroying the fundamental tenets of his rhetorical mode and re-establishing the critical norms of Horace and the Roman rhetoricians. Gascoigne, Puttenham, Webbe, and Jonson did not descend as critics from the writers of the late classical period—from Origen, Julian, and Plotinus—but looked instead to the writers of an earlier age. They set up the basis of what we call neoclassicism today and succeeded so well in their efforts that we no longer recognize the allegorical tradition as classical and think of the Romantics, who revived the allegorical mode, as more original than they were.

It is not the purpose of this chapter to elucidate in detail the various theories of poetry held by men like Puttenham, Jonson, and Sidney. This has already been done by others, in particular by Wesley Trimpi in *Ben Jonson's Poems* (1962) and several writers on Sidney. Rather, I will try to show how these writers *as a group* reversed the basic axioms of allegorical rhetoric, for my concern is not with the new order but with the dying allegorical tradition. Second, I will explain how the reactions of these critics to Spenser's language manifested their practical rejection of his type of poetry. Finally I will make a few suggestions about Sidney and the Metaphysical Poets, who do not exactly belong in either camp. A theorist of Sidney's kind or a poet like John Donne would not really please a strict neoclassicist like Ben Jonson, but they would not agree with Lodge or Harington either. They represent a middle position—the transitional phase from one kind of poetry to another, from that of the Renaissance to that of the Restoration.

A brief résumé of the theory behind allegory will help to clarify the following discussion. The allegorical poet served the truth which he had received under inspiration, and this truth exercised the primary operative control over his rhetoric. He did not really cater to his audience but tried to preserve his truth intact and communicate it to those capable of understanding it. This requirement forced him to deal with two different audiences: the many who could never accept his revelation and the few who could. He had, therefore, simultaneously to reveal and not to reveal his truth, and for this double purpose he cloaked his truth in the veils of allegory. The many reacted with pleasure to his symbolic tales, and the few knew how to interpret them. It was this rhetorical mode which men like Jonson destroyed because they started from an utterly different position.

Critics of such diverse sorts as Sidney, Webbe, Puttenham, and Jonson all concurred in saying that the poet was a maker. In Puttenham's phrase, "The very Poet makes and contriues out of his owne braine, both the verse and matter of his poeme" (*Arte* 1. 1). The poet is a master craftsman who, like God, makes worlds out of nothing. But if the poet creates both the matter and the form of his poetry, one can no longer apply to his work conceptions of verity. He makes objects; he does not communicate truth. So here, at the very basis of their poetics, Spenser's contemporaries differ radically from him. They begin not with truth but with the fact of making. As Sidney says of the poet, "he nothing affirmeth, and therefore never lieth."[1] Allegorical critics often used this same argument but purely for polemical purposes. In actual fact the allegorical poets habitually based their creations on historical events, personal or public, which they

[1] *Defence* F3. 29.

molded into the cosmic truth of myth. They revealed the deeper truth of history and served that truth. In contrast Sidney and Puttenham took this old adage very seriously. The poet affirmed nothing; he made things.

This cleavage between the two groups of critics shows itself still more clearly in their attitudes toward the poet's inspiration. For an allegorical critic like Thomas Lodge, the poet's invocation to the Muses represented a serious appeal for divine aid:

> Whereas the poets were sayde to call for the Muses helpe, ther mening was no other, as Iodocus Badius reporteth, but to call for heauenly inspiration from aboue to direct theyr endauors.

The poet needed divine aid to express a divine truth. But, if the poet made worlds out of his own brain, he obviously did not need the Muses. Trimpi has shown how Ben Jonson burlesqued the standard invocation to the Muses and claimed instead that he wrote by his "owne true fire" (*Forrest* 10. 29).[2] Similarly, the influential Ramists, though they did not think of the poet as a maker, agreed that the invocation to the Muses was a mere figure of speech, which Abraham Fraunce classed under Apostrophe. Sidney considered the invocation to be the poet's way of indicating that what he made was fiction and not truth.[3] None of these writers could take the invocation seriously, and thus at one blow they pulled down the temple of allegory. If the poet does not receive divine truth, he no longer possesses a special kind of truth beyond ordinary human comprehension and has no justification for concealing it. Consequently, his whole rhetorical mode collapses. With divine truth the veils of allegory seem quite necessary; without it, they appear superfluous and give the impression that the poet has deliberately adopted an inflated form of speech.

Not all the critics were as decisive as Sidney in rejecting divine

[2] For the Lodge quotation see G. G. Smith, 1: 72; Wesley Trimpi, *Ben Jonson's Poems* (Stanford, 1962), p. 97.

[3] Abraham Fraunce, *The Arcadian Rhetorike*, ed. Ethel Seaton (Oxford, 1950), 1. 30; for Sidney, see *Defence* F3. 29.

inspiration. Puttenham allowed for it in some cases but did not consider it required for all poetry, and Jonson ascribed the origins of poesy to heaven. Webbe actually quoted Spenser on divine inspiration.[4] But even here the emphasis was radically different. Jonson and Webbe saw this divinity in Horatian terms. The poet's ability to make came from heaven more than any truth he might try to express. For them divine inspiration meant the poetic genius and could be represented by the old phrase: "*Orator fit, poeta nascitur.*" The poet, "raunging within the Zodiack of his owne wit," astonished his audience and revealed his personal genius.[5]

The shift from divine truth to poetic genius in turn occasioned a reappraisal of the relationship between the poet and his art. The allegorist had made the highest possible claims for the art of poetry, but he could regard the poet himself in humble terms. In his Prologues Spenser constantly demeans his own abilities. He asks the Muses for help because his theme surpasses his own capacity.[6] The incipient neoclassicists, on the other hand, reverse this relationship. They exalt the poet but (except for Sidney) do not make any extravagant claims for his art. Poetry may mold the morals and manners of men, but it carries no cosmological message. It may exist only for entertainment, as Puttenham recognizes.[7] Generally, though, the critics maintained the double Horatian ends for poetry: profit and delight. They were by no means agreed that poetry must do both all the time, as Sidney thought.[8] Now an art which can merely entertain has completely lost its superhuman luster. Poetry no longer reveals to man his deeper nature. But for the poet, on the other hand, these critics made very strong claims. Poetry demonstrated one's unique accomplishments and became the medium of personal

[4] *Arte* 1. 1; for Jonson see *Discoveries* HS8: 636-37; for Webbe, see Smith, 1: 232.
[5] *Defence* F3. 8.
[6] *FQ* 1. Pro. 2.
[7] *Arte* 1. 10.
[8] *Defence* F3. 9.

fame. The poet dazzled men by his wit. As Gascoigne remarks, poetry depends upon invention, which must have in it *aliquid salis*, "some good and fine deuise, shewing the quicke capacitie of a writer." Or in the traditional phrase used by Jonson and Puttenham, a poet's style images his mind.[9] It follows that one's judgments about a poem manifest a personal estimation of the writer. The poet magnifies himself through his poetry and so achieves enduring fame.

These critics cannot agree, however, to whom the poet reveals his wit. Sidney and the Ramists envisage a popular audience for the poet. For Sidney this wide audience is absolutely necessary to his argument. The philosopher teaches morality to a limited circle, but the poet stirs up the multitude to moral action. Ramus treats the whole question with a contempt worthy of his attitude (he considered poetry appropriate to small boys) and argues that the prudential method or in medias res technique of the poet exists solely for the vulgar masses, the beast with many heads.[10] The other critics limited the poet's audience to an elite. Jonson equals Boccaccio in his contempt for the unlearned, and Puttenham, like Spenser, appeals to a courtly audience. These critics approach more closely the allegorist's familiar distinction between the few and the many, but the similarity is only superficial. Actually, Jonson is closer to Sidney than to Spenser because, like Sidney, he allows the audience a considerable control over the poet's style, and poetry once more enters the public forum of the orator. In this sense it makes little difference whether the poet addresses a small or large throng because in both cases he must work *within* their commonplaces, unlike the allegorist who serves truth first. The gulf between the two approaches could not be greater.

This matter of audience control appears most clearly in the discussion of invention. Gascoigne advises his friend to avoid the

[9] For Gascoigne, see Smith, 1: 47; *Discoveries* HS8. 625 (Jonson is speaking of language in general); *Arte* 3. 5.
[10] *Ramus*, pp. 283, 253.

trite and obvious. The poet must not bore his audience, but, in contrast to the allegorical poet, his presentation of the unsual is determined not by his truth but by the previous experience of the audience. In 1575 a poet could not praise a woman for her crystal eye or cherry lip, though he could have done so in the past. His inventions depend upon current fashion.[11] Jonson repeats Hoskyns' recommendation and thinks that the poet should consider both his order and his audience when he invents. The artificer must speak to the capacity of his hearers.[12]

Along with audience control poetry quite naturally enters into a close alliance with oratory, a union which an allegorist could never allow. Webbe remarks that rhetorical elocution and poetry are twins by birth and of the same descent. Or as Jonson puts the famous Ciceronian phrase, "The *Poet* is the neerest Borderer upon the Orator."[13] The Ramists went further and classed poetry as a branch of rhetoric,[14] but Jonson would not have accepted such a statement. Nevertheless, to Drummond he suggests Quintilian as a good verse critic, and he uses Hoskyns, a rhetorical critic who depends upon a whole list of rhetoricians: Aristotle, Hermogenes, Quintilian, Demosthenes, Cicero, Sturmius, and Talaeus.[15] Webbe uses Talaeus, and Hoskyns claims that Sidney translated the first two books of Aristotle's *Rhetoric*.[16] These critics look to the rhetoricians for their theories and to that most rhetorical of poetic critics, Horace, whom Webbe summarized and Jonson translated.

This oratorical viewpoint appears in a number of ways. For Puttenham the figures of sense (metaphor, allegory, and the like) are common to both the orator and the poet. He distinguishes the poet by giving him the auricular figures, those which affect one's

[11] In Smith, 1: 48.

[12] *Discoveries* HS8. 629-30; Hoskyns, *Directions for Speech and Style*, ed. Hoyt Hudson (Princeton, 1925), p. 4.

[13] For Webbe, see Smith, 1: 228; *Discoveries* HS8. 640.

[14] *Ramus*, p. 189.

[15] *Conversations* in Herford and Simpson, vol. 1. 132. Hereafter referred to as HS1. Hoskyns gives the list in his Dedicatory Letter.

[16] For Webbe, see Smith, 1: 280; Hoskyns, p. 41.

hearing without altering one's understanding.[17] The allegorical critic, while he likewise stressed the oral nature of poetry, saw rather in the poet's use of the sensible figures the peculiar mark of his art. The poet introduced his audience into a different thought-mode through his use of extended metaphor. For Puttenham no essential difference in psychological approach exists between the orator and the poet. Likewise Puttenham devotes a long chapter to decorum, a Horatian notion. By his examples decorum is defined as the poet's social awareness, his instinctive recognition of his peculiar audience, the requirements of his theme, the time and place. In other words, decorum includes all the considerations an orator must bear in mind when he gives a particular speech. Neither decorum nor an appeal to sound, of course, was foreign to the allegorical critic, but he did not have to give them so much emphasis.

A more significant manifestation of the oratorical viewpoint was the demand for perspicuity in language. The poet, since he depends upon his audience, must make himself clear to them, whether he is addressing an elite group or a popular congregation. Obscurity has no justification for itself, and Boccaccio's long defense of it would not have pleased Puttenham or Jonson. It was by this rubric that all these critics rejected Spenser's experiments with language in *The Shepheardes Calender*, a complex question which we will discuss at length in the next section. At present it suffices to say that the need for perspicuity and normal language formed a part of a larger principle, the Horatian idea that the poet should conceal his art and appear natural to his audience. Puttenham, Jonson, and Webbe all subscribe to this. The purpose of this concealment is again a matter of audience accommodation. As Webbe says, "neyther let him [the poet] so pollish his works but that euery one for the basenesse thereof may think to make as good."[18] Any orator knows that he must not put on airs before his public because they are his judges and he must please

17 *Arte* 3. 10.
18 Rule 53 in Webbe's codification of the *Ars poetica*. In Smith, 1: 390. Or see especially Puttenham's long chapter (*Arte* 3. 25).

them. Or as Puttenham says of decorum, the writer selects his words and figures but the learned decide whether he has succeeded or not. The audience judges, not the poet, even when the judges within that audience are limited to other poets, as Jonson contends.[19]

Given this close affinity between poetry and oratory, these critics had to find some way to distinguish the two arts and chose, appropriately enough, a mechanical means. Poetry is written in verse, oratory is not. Ramus and his disciple Abraham Fraunce accept this distinction, so do the regular critics: Webbe, Puttenham, and Jonson.[20] To use Jonson's explanation:

> The *Poet* is the neerest Borderer upon the Orator, and expresseth all his vertues, though he be tyed more to numbers; is his equall in ornament, and above him in his strengths.

Such a distinction without any metaphysics befits the craftsman's concern with the poetic object, with the thing made. Along with it go elaborate rules for versification in Webbe, Puttenham, and also Gascoigne. Puttenham alone suggests a kind of rationale for verse in itself. It consists in a kind of musical proportion, which imitates the proportion found everywhere in the material world. "All things stand by proportion" (*Arte* 2. 1), and God made the world by number, measure, and tune. The allegorist had identified poetry with the cosmos through its use of sensible figures; Puttenham would do so by its rhythms.

Among these critics Sidney held out and refused to identify poetry with metrical speech, though for his own reasons. In Sidney's view the poet differs from the orator as one without a subject matter differs from one bound to a subject. The poet creates; the orator serves his matter, which is persuasion. On verse Sidney makes the same remarks as does an allegorical critic like Harington. Meter and rhyme delight the ear and memorialize the poet's

---

[19] *Arte* 3. 23; *Discoveries* HS8. 642.
[20] *Ramus*, p. 282; for Webbe, see Smith, 1: 248; *Arte* 1. 1; 2.1; *Discoveries* HS8. 635, 640.

idea within the mind.[21] As Harington says, verse preserves truth
in the way in which we use jingles:

> Another cause why they wrote in verse was conseruation of
> the memorie of their precepts, as we see yet the generall rules
> almost of euerie art, not so much as husbandrie, but they are
> oftner recited and better remembered in verse then in prose.

It is here that the craftsmen's concern for verse as a thing in
itself highlights a basic deficiency in allegorical theory. For Harington verse has the same effects on a hearer as does an allegorical
figure: it strengthens the memory and delights. The allegorist
regards verse as a powerful instrument by which he can intensify
the psychological reactions which he wishes to stimulate in his
audience. It is thus a logical extension of his figural mode into the
ordering of his words. But this reduplication of functions, even
though correct in both instances, demonstrates the failure of the
allegorist to recognize rhythmic speech as something sufficiently
distinct from figured language. Puttenham would not make such
an equation. The allegorist really had no need for verse, though
an allegorical poet like Spenser might experiment widely in verse
forms. Spenser thought of Xenophon's *Cyropaedia* as allegory,
though it was written in prose,[22] and the allegorical apologists
never tired of saying that mere rhymers and versifiers were not
poets. Since the allegorist had no absolute need for verse, he
could not explain the almost universal feeling (at least in the
West) that a rhythmic pattern is essential to poetry. Puttenham
with his sketchy explanation at least tried to understand this.
Rhythmic speech creates a series of musical proportions, as necessary to the ear as images are to the eye. Both figured language
and rhythmic speech are essential to poetry as an oral art, and
both groups of critics—the allegorists and the craftsmen—agreed
that poetry was oral.

Allegory itself was not ignored by the oratorical critics, but

[21] *Defence* F3. 27-28; Harington in Smith, 2: 203.
[22] Letter to Raleigh.

it was relegated to a minor role. Gascoigne considered it to be merely one kind of invention, one way in which the poet could reveal his wit. Judith Dundas has recently developed Gascoigne's equation of allegory with wit in a provocative article: "Allegory as a Form of Wit."[23] Actually, her title should be reversed, for wit is the historical descendant of allegory, as we shall see, an afterglow without the metaphysics, practiced by the "metaphysicals." Puttenham and the Ramists located allegory rather among the figures of speech. It might be the "chief ringleader and captaine of all other figures" (*Arte* 3. 18), as it was in Sherry, and Puttenham can praise it for its courtliness or the Ramists can heap honors upon metaphor, but in all cases allegory has ceased to be synonymous with poetry.[24] It has been sent back to the rhetorical handbooks, not to escape for two hundred years.

What happened at the end of the sixteenth century was a shift from a Platonic, metaphysical conception of the poetic art to a craftsmanlike concern for the finished product—without the metaphysics. Or in rhetorical terms, one can characterize the change by saying that poetry moved from a prophetic mode into the orator's normal mode. Poetry no longer stirred men's memories and recalled to them their true natures; it pleased their minds. It did not change men's lives and create new thought-modes, it informed one's manners and morals. One example epitomizes this change. Ben Jonson confessed to Drummond that he wrote his poetry in prose first and then adapted his phrases to meter and rhyme.[25] That is, he gave measured utterance to rational discourse. He had no visions, no dreams. The age of reason was beginning. Bacon was championing the experimental sciences, and the Ramists were gradually destroying the aural-oral mode altogether. As Ong has shown, Ramus replaced

[23] Gascoigne in Smith, 1: 48. Judith Dundas' article appears in *Studies in the Renaissance*, 11 (1964): 223-33.
[24] Fraunce praises metaphor over all the tropes (*Arcadian Rhetorike*, 1. 7).
[25] *Conversations* HS1. 143.

the allegorical figures of mental processes with spatial diagrams.[26] Allegorical poetry could hardly survive such a change. In this context these craftsmen performed a very necessary function, for they unconsciously devised a way for poetry to survive the rise of science, the worship of reason, and the final disappearance of oral culture. As rhymed reason with few pretensions, poetry could wait for the time when men would want to dream again.

II

This revolution manifested itself on the practical level in the critics' reactions to Spenser's poetic diction. In *The Shepheardes Calender* Spenser deliberately used a specialized vocabulary, made up of archaisms and dialect terms. His experiment had some influence on contemporary writers but received uniform rejection from that group of critics which we have called neoclassical or, perhaps better, oratorical. They opposed his peculiar language either by explicit statements or by the enunciation of general principles. Scholars like R. F. Jones in his *Triumph of the English Language* (Stanford, 1953) have already discussed exhaustively the particular problem involved in Spenser's experiment, i.e., the amplification of the English language. Our concern is otherwise. The critics' opposition to Spenser's language signifies the change in attitude which was occurring. Ultimately, they attacked Spenser's poetic diction because they wanted poetry to be perspicuous, an orator's requirement which extended to more than a poet's choice of words. It excluded allegory itself, in the traditional form which Spenser used. My task here will be, first, to show why Spenser could create a poetic diction; second, the reactions of the oratorical critics; and third, the reasons for their judgments and their implications for allegory.

Nothing could be more natural than for Spenser to create an archaized poetic diction. It was a commonplace among the critics, one which E. K. and Jonson both repeat, that archaic

[26] *Ramus*, p. 91.

terms lend a gravity and dignity to poetic discourse, an air of antiquity borrowed from an olden time.[27] As such, they corresponded perfectly to Spenser's objectives as an allegorical poet: to stimulate in his audience a depth recall, to make men remember their own true natures. Moreover, Cicero had long ago observed the similarity between archaic language and metaphor, which forms the basis of allegorical discourse.[28] They are both *departures* from the normal modes of human expression. In this sense all the figures of speech are abuses of the idiom, ways in which a speaker can lend a strangeness and brilliance to his discourse. It follows that a continued allegory (to use Spenser's phrase) represents a total variation from idiomatic expression, a variation which signifies the unique kind of thought-mode which the poet wishes to create in his auditors. What could be simpler than to extend this variation to the words themselves? Stephen Hawes had already combined an aureate diction with his allegories. One can conclude that Spenser created a poetic diction, not simply because he wished to amplify the language of poetry, but also because such a specialized language suited his purposes. If obscurity resulted from his choice of words, all the better. The allegorist never wished to reveal truth naked but cloaked her about with darkness.

As one might expect, the oratorical critics could not accept Spenser's daring language. Here they all fall into line, whatever their differences: Sidney, Webbe, Fraunce, Puttenham, and Jonson. They reveal their dislike, however, in different ways. Sidney has the weakest argument—for once. He considers archaisms foreign to the tradition of pastoral poetry.[29] Taken literally, this statement is simply wrong. Sidney cites Theocritus as an authority for his position, but Theocritus used both archaisms and dialect terms, and this fact was known in the Renaissance. Taken

[27] Letter to Harvey; *Discoveries* HS8. 622.
[28] *De oratore* 3. 43. 170.
[29] *Defence* F3. 37.

in another way, the argument makes sense. Pastorals were written in the low style, and the conventional definitions of the low style, being drawn from oratorical handbooks, did not allow for archaisms. Richard Sherry says that the low style "is lette downe euen to the mooste vsed custume of pure and clere speakyng." Wilson has a similar definition.[30] The facts of the poetic tradition are against Sidney, particularly when one thinks of English pastoral writers like Turbervile, but the oratorical norms for the low style support his case.

Abraham Fraunce argues more subtly, for, when he selects quotations from Spenser, he simply avoids the noticeably archaized or dialect passages from the *Calender*. Someone who read the *Arcadian Rhetorike* would think that Spenser had the same language as Sidney. Fraunce never commits himself openly; he does not have to. No Ramist could tolerate obscurity anywhere.[31]

Puttenham provides the general rubric which includes Sidney's specific objections. Paraphrasing a passage from Wilson's *Arte of Rhetorike*, he says of language: "This part in our maker or Poet must be heedyly looked vnto, that it be naturall, pure, and the most vsuall of all his countrey" (3. 4).[32] He goes on to narrow speech to a forty-mile area around London and explicitly rejects the use of terms from the professions, dialect words, and archaisms. On the latter his comment reads like a direct refutation of E. K., who had suggested that Spenser picked up his archaic words from his reading of the older English poets: "Our maker therfore at these dayes shall not follow *Piers plowman* nor *Gower* nor *Lydgate* nor yet *Chaucer*, for their language is now out of vse with vs." Puttenham wants the poet to use a language clear to any reasonably educated audience. Archaisms

---

30 Richard Sherry, A *Treatise of Schemes & Tropes* (London, 1550), fB iv^r; Wilson, *Arte of Rhetorike*, f86^v.

31 *Ramus*, p. 284.

32 Wilson, f 1^v – 2^r; 82^v – 83^r.

and dialect terms, therefore, cannot be allowed, since they are not generally intelligible. Sensible advice—for an orator. Cicero said it long before.[33]

Jonson both explains this general principle and points out Spenser as an offender:[34]

> Spenser in affecting the Ancients, writ no Language.
>
> .   .   .   .
> Custom is the most certaine Mistresse of Language, as the publicke stampe makes the current money. But wee must not be too frequent with the mint, every day coyning. Nor fetch words from the extreme and utmost ages; since the chiefe vertue of a style is perspicuitie, and nothing so vitious in it, as to need an Interpreter.

If Spenser had been perspicuous, he would not have needed E. K. Webbe, enthusiastic Spenserian though he is, nevertheless says much the same thing and indicates his authority—Horace.[35]

Jonson here exposes the wider implications of this Horatian axiom, which can be applied not only to Spenser's language but to the allegorical form itself. No poetry should need an interpreter, and Jonson dryly remarks elsewhere that Spenser had to explain his *Faerie Queene* in a letter to Raleigh. Of allegory he says that a writer should not continue it too long, "lest either wee make our selves obscure, or fall into affectation, which is childish."[36] Spenser drew out his allegory over six books and some 30,000 lines.

The other critics similarly noted the obscurity in Spenser's allegory. William Webbe confessed that he could not understand parts of *The Shepheardes Calender*,[37] despite E. K.'s commentary. Gabriel Harvey in effect admitted the label, though he regarded it positively. He praised one of Spenser's poems because it was "a degree or two at the leaste, aboue the reache, and

---

[33] Cicero *De oratore* 3. 10. 38-39.
[34] *Discoveries* HS8. 618, 622.
[35] Smith, 1: 291 (Rule 7).
[36] *Conversations* HS1. 132; *Discoveries* HS8. 625.
[37] Smith, 1: 264.

compasse of a common Schollers capacitie."[38] While Sidney does not make any specific statement, he could hardly regard a poem like *The Faerie Queene* as popular philosophy.

The charge of obscurity could sometimes imply a further charge of moral obliquity on the part of the poet. Samuel Daniel considered the use of strange words and,foreign terms little worse than self-conceit, a deliberate affectation of singularity and a distrust of the English language.[39] Marston, who praised *The Faerie Queene*, still has his satirist exclaim:

> . . . This affectation,
> To speake beyond mens apprehension,
> How Apish tis. When all in fusten sute
> Is cloth'd a huge *nothing*, all for repute
> Of profound knowledge, when profoundnes knowes
> There's nought contain'd, but only seeming showes.
>
> [*Scourge* 9. 66-71]

Jonson likewise associated affectation with obscurity. Rhetorically, these judgments again presuppose an audience situation in which a poet like Spenser would inevitably sound affected, betraying a certain insincerity. He would appear to value manner over matter, or, in Milton's phrase, he would make "verbal curiosities the end."[40] To create confidence in such a situation, a speaker must talk in the manner of the ordinary man. He must conceal his art, not display it.

To such a demand what could Spenser have said? With his poetic diction, complicated stanza forms, and difficult allegory, he everywhere drew attention to his art as art. All he could hope was that some critic might say to him what Antigenidas the flute player said to his pupil when the audience received his performance coldly: "Play for me and for the Muses" (*Brutus* 49. 187). By the standards of oratory he could say nothing. In the new

---

[38] From *Three Proper and Wittie, Familiar Letters*, in the Variorum Spenser, *Prose Works*, p. 471.

[39] See the last two paragraphs of A *Defence of Ryme*.

[40] *Discoveries* HS8. 625; *Reason of Church Government*, 2: 236 in the Columbia Edition of the *Works* (New York, 1931), vol. 3. part 1.

order there was no room for his kind of allegory, much less for his poetic diction. It is not surprising that editions of *The Faerie Queene* became infrequent after 1620. Allegory was dead. The success of this revolution can already be seen in miniature in E. K.'s defense of *The Shepheardes Calender*. E. K. failed in his argument for Spenser's language experiments largely because he was arguing from the wrong frame of reference. His authorities were Horace, Cicero, and perhaps Quintilian, none of whom could have countenanced Spenser's poetic diction. But let us look at his arguments in some detail.

His major contention—that the poet had to amplify the vocabulary of the vernacular—was a cliché by 1579. E. K. thought that the use of archaisms achieved this purpose better than foreign words, a defensible position. There were recognized arguments for and against this idea, and E. K. employed one of them. His first argument likewise had some substance. He borrowed Turbervile's old claim that archaic language suited the speakers of an eclogue. This was a question of decorum, and Turbervile himself began his discussion of the matter appropriately enough with the first verses of Horace's *Ars poetica*. It was reasonable to contend that rustics should use outmoded terms. Over two hundred years later Coleridge caught Wordsworth doing the same thing.[41] But decorum, as Puttenham showed, is a complex matter, subject to varying interpretations, and one could, therefore, attack Spenser by the same principle. Sidney's argument is a good example. For reasons of decorum he objects to archaized language in the eclogue. Low characters require a low style, which by definition does not allow for archaic words. In any case E. K. at least had some reasonable arguments, though all of them admitted serious doubt.

It is on the general level that E. K.'s argument breaks down. Here he repeats the Ciceronian theory that archaic words lend

---

[41] George Turbervile in his translation of Mantuan's *Eglogs* (London, 1567), fAiv^r. For Coleridge, see the *Biographia Literaria*, 17, pp. 536-37 in the *Portable Coleridge*, ed. I. A. Richards (New York, 1961).

gravity and dignity to a composition. Jonson says exactly the same thing, as does Quintilian.[42] What E. K. tries to get around is the principle of perspicuity, which controls this argument and which all these critics assume. A poet may use archaic words, so long as they do not impede communication with his audience. The auditor must understand the work initially, at least on a superficial level, a criterion applicable both to poetry and to the law courts. Puttenham, though he excludes any archaizing at all, argues from the same principle.

From this general criterion one derives two rules of practice: (1) the writer must avoid archaic words which are really obsolete, i.e., no longer intelligible, (2) he must not use too many archaisms in any single passage. Jonson presents these rules in the passage quoted earlier, borrowing his phraseology from Horace.[43] E. K. obviously worried about them too. He half admitted that Spenser violated the first rule:

> And firste of the wordes to speake, I graunt they
> be something hard, and of most men vnused . . .
> such olde and obsolete wordes . . . old and
> vnwonted words . . . English words, as haue ben
> long time out of vse and almost cleane dishcrited.

He defended Spenser on the second rule, as have some of Spenser's modern supporters, who have painstakingly counted all the archaisms in the *Calender*.[44] Unfortunately, number totals do not pass Ben Jonson's simple and practical test. Does the reader of Spenser need an interpreter or not? E. K.'s massive commentary gives the answer and defeats his own argument. E. K. could not really defend Spenser this way, and he did not suc-

---

[42] For Quintilian, see *Institutio oratoria* 8. 3. 24f.

[43] Horace *Ars poetica* 46-62.

[44] E. K. remarks in his Letter to Harvey: "Yet nether euery where must old words be stuffed in, nor the commen Dialecte and maner of speaking so corrupted therby, that as in old buildings it seme disorderly and ruinous." For a summary of the modern arguments, see Appendix IV in the Variorum *Minor Poems*, vol. 1.

ceed in convincing anyone but Webbe, who was not exactly the most intelligent man of the period.[45] It is ironic and also typical of the age that Spenser moved in a circle of friends who had very different approaches to the poetic art. Harvey was a Ramist, E. K. belonged to the oratorical school of critics, and Sidney had his own unique point of view. None of them really agreed with Edmund Spenser, but then none of them agreed exactly with each other. They well represent the transitional character of the period, going off in all directions. But Sidney most truly epitomized the transition. Brilliant and original, he belonged neither among the allegorists nor among the orators, and, therefore, his theories anticipate the metaphysical poets in this respect, that they too belonged nowhere. It is to them that we must now turn.

III

We have already discussed Sidney insofar as his theories opposed the traditional allegorical conceptions of the poet's role, and basically that is where he belongs—in the oratorical camp. But, unlike Ben Jonson, he managed to bridge the gulf separating the orator from the allegorist and made in his *Defence* high claims both for the poet and for his art, something neither Spenser nor Jonson could have done. The tone of his rhetoric suggested the exalted claims for the poetic art made by the allegorist, a purpose which he accomplished by borrowing most of the clichés of allegorical criticism, though he came up with very different conclusions. The manner in which he talks about the word *vates* and the poetic genius, for example, convinces his audience that poetry is divinely inspired, despite his explicit denial of the idea later on.[46] He devised an approach which included both viewpoints on poetry and as such anticipated the

---

[45] Webbe gives E. K.'s arguments. See Smith, 1: 263.
[46] *Defence* F3. 34.

Romantics, who likewise exalted the poetic genius and yet revived many notions common to allegorical criticism.

We have already reviewed some of the commonplaces he shares with the allegorical critics. He does not consider verse essential to poetry, and he has the same explanation for its function: it delights the hearer and impresses his memory. Discussing Christ's parables, he repeats what Peacham said of the figure *allegoria:* they would "more constantly as it were, inhabit both the memorie and judgement."[47] He likes Plato best of the philosophers, and we have seen how the allegorists instinctively looked to Plato for a philosophical rationale for their art. He shares with Spenser the Platonic notion that the excellence of a work is found rather in its idea or "fore conceit" than in itself.[48] He argues that Xenophon's Cyrus both surpasses any of Nature's productions and has within itself more vitality. It can create other Cyruses through human imitation. This line of reasoning closely resembles the discussion of euhemeristic myth in an earlier chapter. The poet makes historical individuals into gods, which in turn become patterns for other human beings to follow. And finally, when he upsets the Aristotelian ladder, he makes the same distinction between poetry and philosophy drawn in late classical times and continued in the allegorical tradition. Philosophy appeals only to the few, while poetry can lead even the vulgar mob to moral action. The Emperor Julian would have agreed.

Despite this array of common viewpoints, Sidney held an essentially alien position, for he drew different conclusions. The last commonplace provides a good example. Both Sidney and Julian believed that poetry could lead the common man to right moral action, but their attitudes toward this fact were at variance. Julian attributes this function to myth more-or-less in passing, for he is more concerned wih its services to the elite:

47 Ibid., p. 15.
48 Ibid., p. 8.

Now I think ordinary men derive benefit enough from the irrational myth which instructs them through symbols alone. But those who are more highly endowed with wisdom will find the truth about the gods helpful. . . .

[*Oration* 5. 170b]

And most of his *Oration* describes just what the "more highly endowed" will learn. Sidney, on the other hand, bases much of his argument on this point. Poetry appeals to all men, young and old, educated and uneducated. He has no interest in any special messages which the poet might have for the few. Poetry surpasses philosophy and history because it creates within an audience real assent to moral positions (if I may borrow Newman's phrase, which he uses for the same purpose).[49] For Sidney the poet functions in a truly prophetic role—he reforms the morals of all the people. But at a price. The prophet, struggling under divine inspiration, could never succeed in his task. Sidney's poet can succeed because in a normal situation he has no divine truth to worry about and, thus, no inner reality which the wise might want to learn. So we come again to the crucial notion of inspiration and Sidney's reinterpretation of it.

Though he discounted any direct inspiration, Sidney brought in the notion by another means. He saw in the poet's ability to make things evidence for man's divinity. Only God and poets can make worlds out of nothing. Thus, he located the divine at the heart of his own poetics. The poet surpasses Nature in his creations and reveals man's superiority to his environment. As he says in the *Defence*:

Neither let it be deemed too sawcy a comparison, to ballance the highest point of mans wit, with the efficacie of nature: but rather give right honor to the heavenly maker of that maker, who having made man to his owne likenes, set him beyond and over all the workes of that second nature, which in nothing he sheweth so much as in Poetry; when with the force of a divine breath, he bringeth things foorth

[49] Chapter 4 in Newman's *A Grammar of Assent* (New York, 1955), especially pp. 76-92.

surpassing her doings: with no small arguments to the in-
credulous of that first accursed fall of *Adam*, since our erected
wit maketh us know what perfection is, and yet our infected
wil keepeth us from reaching unto it.

The poet reveals to man a perfect world and a perfect humanity,
his version of what once existed at the beginning of time. He,
therefore, bears witness to man's divinity, to the Man made in
the image of God. The result in his audience is similar. The
architectonic end of all the arts is praxis—doing well besides
knowing well. The poet alone accomplishes this end, by creating a visionary paradise where ideal men think and act well. His
vision instructs and his images move his audience to live the
vision—to make it real to the extent that they are able. Or as
Sidney puts it, "the finall end is, to lead and draw us to as high
a perfection, as our degenerate soules made worse by their clay-
lodgings, can be capable of."[50]

In more philosophical terms the allegorists made substantially the same claim. The poet practised anamnesis; he recalled
to man what in fact he had once experienced. The allegorists,
therefore, had a more objective conception of the poet's function. Sidney's poet wove ideal images out of nothing; they had
no basis in reality, though they could affect it. The allegorists
went further. The poet's fictions reflected a true situation. The
soul recalled through vision its actual paradisic state. It perceived the ideas in the Divine Mind and wove this revelation
into a figured discourse which would re-create the same vision in
other people. The vision could be transferred because all men
had once experienced it and needed only a powerful stimulus to
draw it out of their deeper memories. This is a more far-reaching
claim, but one dependent upon the theory of divine inspiration.
Without a direct channel to the divinity, the poet could not
maintain for himself more than Sidney does. Sidney kept what
he could of the old traditions.

He may have kept too much, for he stuffs into his peroration

[50] *Defence* F3. 8,11.

a remark which could seriously upset his argument. He exhorts his audience "To beleeue with me, that there are many misteries contained in *Poetrie*, which of purpose were written darkly, least by prophane wits it should be abused."[51] That is, poetry is allegory which is written for an elite and which cloaks truth from the multitude. He presents this as his own belief, but, if he seriously maintained this position, his whole argument could come into question. In what sense would the poet be a "populer *Philosopher*,"[52] if he concealed truth from the populace? Worse, how can the poet cloak truth when he neither affirms or denies? This notion of truth is crucial because Sidney's refutation of Aristotle depends upon the exclusion of truth from poetry. Otherwise, he loses the argument, because the Aristotelian ladder was originally designed to elevate philosophy as abstract truth over poetry as concrete truth. A possible explanation for this comment does exist within the bounds of Sidney's argument, but he does not make it at all explicit.

In his discussion of the three kinds of poetry, Sidney includes two kinds in which the poet does not choose to make his own matter but binds himself instead to a particular subject either in philosophy or in theology. In such a situation a poet is controlled by his subject matter as much as an astronomer, philosopher, or historian is by his. The notion of truth, therefore, arises once more, because a poet can be wrong about the secrets of nature just as a historian can be wrong about his facts or an astronomer about stellar movements. So here in philosophical and theological poetry Sidney's maker could well cloak truth from the multitude, and he would be concealing the very same kind of truths which the allegorist protected. If this explanation is at all valid, it puts Sidney much closer to the allegorists than he usually appears to be. But he backs away from the position as much as possible. He is not certain that versified philosophy should be called poetry precisely because the poet is bound to his

---

[51] Ibid., p. 45.
[52] Ibid., p. 16.

subject matter and does not have freedom to invent, and he puts all his emphasis on the third kind of poetry, where the writer makes up his own matter.[53] He does not apply the same criticism to theological poetry, presumably because the infinite nature of God allows the poet freedom of invention and because he believes that the poets of the Bible were inspired by the Holy Ghost. In any case the most one can say is that Sidney allows for allegory as one kind of invention, which is what Gascoigne says. The notion of truth and the allegorical veil apply only to some poems, and those are a small number.

As the foregoing discussion has shown, Sidney is a difficult man to classify. True to his theory of genius, he remains a little too witty for the systematizer. He begins his *Apology* with an anecdote about a certain Pugliano, who so overpraised horsemanship that he almost convinced Sidney to become a horse. Sidney implies that he will do the same for poetry, so all his high praise cannot be taken completely seriously. He waxes enthusiastic over his craft and makes extravagant claims for it, just as Pugliano does for horsemanship. The strain of humor which runs through the oration keeps his audience aware of this self-conscious irony. Ultimately, one must say that Sidney escapes any simple classification. His oration is too witty and includes too many diverse elements. Or one might say that Sidney had wit enough to combine both worlds: that of Spenser and that of Jonson.

IV

Sidney was not alone in his middle position. A metaphysical poet like John Donne also had the wit to write a kind of poetry obedient neither to the norms of a Jonson or Puttenham nor to the conceptions of a Lodge or Harington. It is outside the scope of this study to cover such a complicated matter in any detail, but some suggestions can be made.

In his *The Proper Wit of Poetry* (1961) George Williamson

[53] Ibid., pp. 9-10.

has already defined with great care the notions of wit which affected Donne's poetry. For his sources Williamson draws upon oratorical critics like Puttenham, Gascoigne, and Hoskyns, a sufficient indication of Donne's relation to the new order. For us it is enough to quote Ben Jonson's epigram:

> Donne, the delight of PHŒBVS, and each Muse,
> Who, to thy one, all other braines refuse;
> Whose euery worke, of thy most earely wit,
> Came forth example, and remaines so, yet:
> Longer a knowing, then most wits doe liue
> [Epigrammes 23]

Donne has received the laurel garland through his wit, producing poetry dependent on no other mind. This is substantially Carew's evaluation in his famous Elegie. In other words, the criteria of the craftsmen or oratorical critics aptly characterize his achievement. Donne himself described poetry as a counterfeit creation, which makes things that are not as though they were,[54] words which would have pleased Puttenham. And in an epistle to Rowland Woodward he compares life to a dream and his poem to a dream image. Allegory had wakened people from the dream of life, but Donne's poetry remains within the dream, the mundane. He created poetry out of nothing—out of his own brains—and his genius easily surpassed that of his contemporaries. He could write allegory when he chose, as in the Anniversaries, but, like Gascoigne, Donne treated allegory as just one form of invention. His Elegies contain no allegory, while every poem of Spenser has an allegorical dimension. Donne does not identify poetry with allegory. Instead poetry proceeds from wit or invention, of which allegory is a variety. But there is another side to his poetry. George Williamson also remarks that many of Donne's witty effects depend upon a violation of decorum,[55] and, as we shall see later, he did not gauge his poetry to the capacity of his hearers. He violated the principle of perspicuity, just as

---

[54] LXXX Sermons (London, 1640), p. 266 (Sermon 26).
[55] Proper Wit of Poetry (Chicago, 1961), pp. 19-20.

Spenser did. Even in the notion of wit, the very basis of seventeenth-century poetry,[56] conceptions existed which approximated rather the allegorists' approach to poetry, and Donne's own work bears the marks.

Cowley's famous definition of wit is essentially Neoplatonic and his analogies to salvation history and the supercelestial world would have pleased a Pico della Mirandola:

> In a true piece of W*it* all things must be,
>   Yet all things there *agree*.
> As in the *Ark*, joyn'd without force or strife,
> All *Creatures* dwelt; all *Creatures* that had *Life*.
>   Or as the *Primitive Forms* of all
>   (If we compare great things with small)
> Which without *Discord* or *Confusion* lie,
> In that strange *Mirror* of the *Deitie*.
>
> [*Of Wit* 57-64]

All things, not *some* or *many*, for the poet must create a unity out of everything, or at least make his audience think that he has. Underlying this definition is the old allegorical notion that every poem both imitated the cosmos and became a world unto itself, an idea which Lewis calls the old confusion of poetry with encyclopedias.[57] The poet tried to create within his work a richness and variety as well as a system of relations which mirrored the plentitude and the ordered relationships which made up the cosmos. Sidney and the craftsmen also considered the poet's creations to be other worlds, golden worlds in Sidney's theory, which surpassed the creations of nature. The poet made more pleasant rivers, trees, and flowers than nature herself could produce, and Arthur Wilson praised Donne for accomplishing just that.[58] But neither Sidney nor the craftsmen ever claimed that the poet's world actually reflected the objective series of relationships which existed in the cosmos. This idea appeared rather in

[56] Ibid., p. 18.

[57] Lewis, *English Literature*, p. 321.

[58] *Upon Mr. J. Donne, and his* Poems, p. 397 in the 1633 edition of Donne's *Poems*.

the *Heptaplus* of Pico della Mirandola and in allegorical commentaries on the epic, which by its greater length could include more things.[59] Donne was acquainted with this idea through his reading of the *Heptaplus*, and Helen Gardner has argued that his later lyrics show a Neoplatonic influence.[60]

Almost any poem of Donne dazzles one by the variety of connections which he makes to a central idea, and this is particularly true of the later lyrics. To take one at random, in *Love's Growth* he relates love successively to grass, the seasons, the quintessence and medicine, the artificial Muse of conventional love poetry, the stars in the firmament, blossoms on a bough, circles in the water, the heavenly spheres—and war taxes. He associates his love implicitly with the cosmos and human history, an association which valorizes both his love and the cosmos: the one by magnifying its relations, the other by centering the world on a positive, personal emotion. His display of extraordinary erudition further contributes to this cosmic effect, for what could a poet of encyclopedic knowledge produce but an encyclopedic poem? Donne's endless subtleties about alchemy, astrology, and the obscure sciences help to convince his audience that he indeed knows everything and that his poems, therefore, contain everything. He has compared his love to so many different things that we are led to believe that he could continue the comparisons ad infinitum; so that a tiny lyric by its density and richness suggests the fullness of creation, the microcosm of the macrocosm. In the *Songs and Sonnets* he intensifies this effect when he links his individual poems by the same principle. He juxtaposes the many contrary attitudes which lovers can take: the libertine of the *Indifferent*, the Platonic lover of the *Relique*, the grieving husband of the *Nocturnall*, as well as the many possible situations in a love affair, extending to several episodes *after* death (the *Apparition* or the *Relique*). The probable arrangement of the poems

59 See Chapman in Smith, 2: 299.
60 John Donne, *Elegies, and the Songs and Sonnets of John Donne*, ed. Helen Gardner (Oxford, 1965), pp. xxx, lix (especially the first footnote).

likewise suggests a cosmic pattern.[61]It imitates the cycle of a day (morning to evening) and the course of love from birth to death. The titles signify this: the *Good-morrow*, the *Sun-Rising*; the *Funeral*, the *Relique*, and the *Dampe*. In its own fashion the *Songs and Sonnets* shares in the cosmic depth and variety of the *Faerie Queene* itself.

One's response to the *Songs and Sonnets* differs significantly, however, from the reactions caused by a poem like *The Faerie Queene*. One admires Spenser's dream, his visionary outlook on things, never before imagined, while one admires the poet of the *Songs and Sonnets*. Shared vision has become personal tribute to the genius and sensibility of Donne, who contrives his own universe of love—out of his own individuality. For all his closeness to the allegorical tradition Donne remains basically the maker and craftsman. He achieves immortality not for his vision but for himself, dreaming, thinking, and feeling. The difference is crucial. Donne relates to Sidney and Puttenham, rather than to Pico, Lodge, or Spenser. The *Anniversaries* are a good example of this difference. They are allegories, for, as Donne said to Jonson, he described in them not Elizabeth Drury, whom he had never met, but "the Idea of a Woman."[62] Here, if anywhere, one would expect to find something close to Spenser, but the effect of these poems is quite different. They immortalize Donne as much as Elizabeth. His presence as a unique person is felt strongly in the allegories. He ends the *First Anniversarie* with an elaborate explanation of why he wrote the poem and concludes that he is the new Moses, delivering the Law to his people. Elizabeth may be his subject, but he draws as much attention to himself.

Even so, neither Puttenham nor Jonson could really allow for his achievement. His poetry depended too much on a Pla-

---

[61] I am referring to the order in the Group I Ms, which Helen Gardner conjectures might have been arranged for publication in 1614. See her edition, pp. lxiv-lxv; lxxxiii.

[62] Quoted by Frank Manley in his edition of the *Anniversaries* (Baltimore, 1963), p. 7.

tonic union-in-diversity and violated the essential stylistic norm of the oratorical critics—that of perspicuity. To unify the unlike, Donne drew upon the language of the professions and the obscure sciences, a practice which Puttenham objected to as much as he did to Spenser's archaic diction, and for the same reason.[63] It unduly limited the poet's audience. A poet like Donne deliberately created difficulties for his auditors. He did not accommodate himself to their capacities. He was as obscurantist as Spenser himself, and he was criticized on the same grounds, both then and later. Jonson's comment is well known: "that Done himself for not being understood would perish";[64] and, according to Wesley Trimpi, he associated Donne's style with that of the archaizing Sallust, a classic type of the obscure. Jasper Mayne agreed with Jonson, though, of course, reversing his judgment. He said of Donne's poetry "that wee are thought wits, when 'tis understood."[65] Donne's printer appealed only to the "Understanders,"[66] and Joseph Hall repeated the substance of Mayne's comment, applying the idea to the *Second Anniuersary*:

> . . . let me wonder at thy flight
> Which long agone had'st lost the vulgar sight
> And now mak'st proud the better eyes, that thay
> Can see thee less'ned in thine aery way.
> [*Harbinger* 23-26]

Both Donne and Spenser were princes of darkness.

Like Sidney, Donne through his wit ultimately escapes classification. He belongs with the craftsmen as a witty maker, but on the crucial matter of audience accommodation he sides with Spenser. Part of this can be attributed to the cult of darkness,

---

[63] *Arte* 3. 4.

[64] *Conversations* HS1. 138.

[65] Trimpi, pp. 3-40. George Williamson gives the quotation from Jasper Mayne in his classic essay on "strong lines," now printed in *Seventeenth Century Contexts* (Chicago, 1961), p. 123. The basic discussion of Donne's coterie audience is now, of course, the opening chapter of Alvarez' *The School of Donne*. Though agreeing in general with his thesis, I would object to his tacit classification of Spenser with Sidney.

[66] *Poems* (London, 1633).

started by Muret and Lipsius in imitation of Seneca and Tacitus, and this movement resembles the allegorical tradition in its taking care to hide unpopular opinions. Moreover, the poet who speaks not from but of the heart courts obscurity because inner truth escapes clear definition or portrayal, especially in a highly educated and intelligent individual like Donne. This likeness to Spenser at the same time indicates the transitional nature of metaphysical poetry. It contained within itself too much of the old tradition to survive the revolution: too much Neoplatonism, too much obscurantism, in effect, too much of the "metaphysics." As Dryden remarked, Donne "perplexes the minds of the fair sex with nice speculations of philosophy, when he should engage their hearts, and entertain them with the softnesses of love."[67] The effects of this revolution can already be seen *within* the metaphysical school—in the poetry of George Herbert.

Herbert has long been considered a metaphysical poet, more or less in the tradition of Donne, but Rosemond Tuve in *A Reading of George Herbert* (1952) has demonstrated that he also was something of an allegorist. He cast his *Temple* in allegorical form and used the traditional metaphors and symbols of the Christian-biblical tradition. He was both metaphysical and an allegorist, and yet he differs significantly from either Donne or Spenser, since his poetry comes much closer to the norm of perspicuity. His style is simple, his wit restrained, and his allegory depends upon popular symbols, unfamiliar to us but well known in the seventeenth century. In fact, he explicitly rejects in his Jordan poems the obscurity of allegory and the excesses of metaphysical wit, regarding the latter correctly as a form of self-glorification:

> Is it no verse, except enchanted groves
> And sudden arbours shadow course-spunne lines?
> Must purling streams refresh a lovers loves?
> Must all be vail'd, while he that reades, divines,
>   Catching the sense at two removes?
>
> [*Jordan* I]

[67] In the Scott-Saintsbury edition of the *Works* (Edinburgh, 1887), 13. 6.

My thoughts began to burnish, sprout, and swell,
Curling with metaphors a plain intention,
Decking the sense, as if it were to sell.

[*Jordan* II]

It was Spenser who combined complicated allegorical landscapes with "course-spunne lines," verses tinged with archaisms and dialect terms. The second description has always been considered an excellent characterization of metaphysical poetry, but Herbert regards its effects as much the same as those of Spenserian allegory: metaphors obscure the plain sense of the text. Herbert came to this attitude through his situation as a Christian preacher in the provinces. He says in the seventh chapter of the *Country Parson* that a preacher "is not witty, or learned, or eloquent, but Holy." The parson must speak from the heart (not of it, as Donne did), honestly and sincerely. Metaphysical wit and allegory would both produce the opposite effect on such an audience. Such devices must be restrained and simplified. Thus, Herbert through his vocation ended up modeling his poetic theory on oratory, as Jonson had done. The norms of the pulpit are the same as those of the rostrum. He labored to conceal his art, and nothing could be more expressive of his method than the figure poems, which Puttenham had advocated. Read aloud, they seem simple, direct speech. Seen on the page, they form an artistic figure, an altar or wings. Herbert more than anyone, perhaps, put into effect the old principle: *ars est celare artem*.

Herbert is a sign of the end. Allegory and its afterglow, the metaphysical style, were rapidly dying. Even Cowley, Donne's most famous successor, tended to use similes where Donne would have used metaphors; that is, he rationalized the relations which he was establishing. He clarified by simplification. Final defeat came with the Restoration, when the neoclassical poets could ignore the old allegorical conceptions completely and shelter themselves under the authority of Aristotle as well as that of Horace, the rhetoricians, and their own writers. As disciples of Aristotle, they tended to use drama as a model for poetry and consequently had to require clarity everywhere, since the audience in a theater, like one in a courtroom or in a church, is unspecialized and cannot puzzle out a text. Here the precepts of the rhetoricians and those of Aristotle coalesce, for it was Aristotle who said: "The perfection of Diction is for it to be at once clear and not mean."[68] The translator of Boileau speaks for them all when he urges poets to imitate Waller and "be, like him, in your expressions, clear."[69]

In the seventeenth century the one significant exception to this general trend was John Milton. In *Paradise Lost* he combined the oratorical and allegorical modes more than Sidney or Donne—one reason, perhaps, why he outshines everyone in the period but Shakespeare and has had such an enormous influence. His style was perspicuous, but his plot was mythic and allegoric, and he believed in divine inspiration. The eighteenth century imitated his clear, high-sounding style, and the Romantics his myth. Solitary and blind, he recovered something of the magic which has made the works of Sophocles and Virgil quasi-eternal. Few are the poets who can be clear and yet profound.

What allegory survived the change was of the simplified, clear type which Herbert used but—after Bunyan—without the profundity of his Christian symbols. Or it might more accurately be said that the term *allegory* became separated from the mythic speech which it originally denoted. Samuel Johnson in the *Rambler* included allegories which in ancient terms would be called moral *exempla*. What could Spenser have made of this title: "The Observance of Sunday Recommended; an Allegory"?[70] He would rather have called the mythologies of Blake and Shelley allegories, and Blake indeed at one time of his life made the same equation. In a Letter to Thomas Butts he called one of his poems an allegory and went on to explain: "Allegory addressed to the

---

[68] *Poetics* 22. 1458a; the translation is by Ingram Bywater in the McKeon edition of the *Basic Works* (New York, 1941).

[69] *Art of Poetry*, 1: 142; in Scott-Saintsbury, vol. 15.

[70] *Rambler* 30 (London, 1824).

Intellectual powers, while it is altogether hidden from the Corporeal Understanding, is My Definition of the Most Sublime Poetry."[71] A late classical critic would have agreed perfectly with this statement. But later in his life he rejected this notion of allegory and separated it from vision, by which he meant what Spenser would call allegory.[72] Coleridge further confused matters, as Angus Fletcher has explained in his study, *Allegory* (1964), in which he distinguishes allegory from symbol, meaning by the word *allegory* something closer to an *exemplum* and using the word *symbol* to denote something more like Spenserian allegory. The confusion has persisted ever since. Ironically, one can say that allegory as a term died just as its meaning was being revived, for the Romantics were myth-makers and allegorists.

[71] *Selected Poetry and Prose of William Blake*, ed. Northrop Frye (New York, 1953), pp. 423-24.
[72] Ibid., p. 386.

Postscript: Some Romantics

> All high poetry is infinite; it is as the first acorn,
> which contained all oaks potentially. Veil after veil
> may be undrawn, and the inmost naked beauty of
> the meaning never exposed.
> [Shelley, *A Defence of Poetry*]

IT HAS BEEN a minor thesis of this book that the Romantics revived allegory in English poetry, and the claim requires some clarification. The present vogue of allegorical criticism stems in great part from Northrop Frye and involves a more or less Romantic attitude toward the old allegory. It might be useful to reverse this perspective and view the Romantics from the standpoint of the Renaissance. The tradition is a long one, extending over two thousand years, and one can move forward or backward in it. Frye began his studies with William Blake, whose comments on vision poetry might have pleased an Alexandrian exegete of the Bible. The links in the chain are often missing, but the allegorists' structuring of the poetic process remains astonishingly consistent, despite the many revolutions in thought and society. Blake may have learned his theories from his friend, Thomas Taylor, himself steeped in the traditions of the late classical period. Whatever the source, the tradition is there. Praise has been given to the Romantics for their originality and their break with the past, but I think higher praise should be given to men like Shelley, who managed to revive mythic poetry in a rationalist age, which itself in large measure had killed the old allegory.

For our purposes it will be sufficient to isolate the two ends of the Romantic spectrum: Wordsworth and Shelley. The former has more affinity to the oratorical tradition than one might expect, while the latter revived allegorical theory almost in toto. Taken together, they show both the closeness and the difference of the Romantics and the Renaissance practitioners of myth.

I
William Wordsworth

Both Wordsworth and Shelley structure the poetic process in the same way, and this structure corresponds point by point to the model used by the Renaissance allegorist. The Romantics vary from each other and differ as a group from the Renaissance theorists in their explanation of this structure. The form remains the same, but the content changes. I will begin with Wordsworth.

In his definition of poetry Wordsworth incorporated the famous fountain analogy, one which Boccaccio had used in a different application but with similar results. Wordsworth identifies the fountain with the poet, whose feelings overflow spontaneously.[1] Boccaccio identifies it with the critic, who reveals fresh water gushing from the flaming globe of poetic myth (GDG 14. 1). The two emphasize the different ends of the poetic act—its origin in the poet and its result within another person—but they choose the same metaphor and, as we shall see, presuppose the same action in both the poet and his auditor. We have already discussed how the allegorical poet re-creates within his audience the same vision which he once experienced. Wordsworth assumes the same scheme but explains it in an eighteenth-century psychological idiom. The poet has a larger imaginative and sympathetic power than other men, and through his poetry he extends the imaginative capability of his readers. A man par-

---

[1] All quotations and paraphrases from Wordsworth are taken from his Preface to the Second Edition of the *Lyrical Ballads* with its supplements. In the Hutchinson-Selincourt edition, pp. 734-51.

ticipates in Wordsworth's emotions when he reads one of his poems. He imitates the experience behind the poem. Wordsworth's explanation, however, significantly changes one's understanding of this structure. Boccaccio's auditor rationalized a poem, struggling with it intellectually to find the vision behind it. He did not look for an imaginative expression of passion. In choosing a current psychological analysis of this structure, Wordsworth has replaced vision with feeling, and the poet is no longer rapt above the spheres.

In the same line Wordsworth emphasizes the spontaneous nature of the poetic act, reviving the theory of divine inspiration in psychological terms. Poetry has a divine origin, and he instinctively associates it with religion,[2] just as the old commentators had thought of myth through analogies with the pagan mysteries. Wordsworth even preserves traces of the old memory theory. His poet does not actually express his emotions on the spot, as Byron did during the Alpine storm. He *recollects* his emotions in tranquillity. Again, Wordsworth gives memory a psychological explanation instead of the old Platonic and metaphysical one. Wordsworth's poet simulates through memory the state of his original emotions and then proceeds to compose. He recalls feeling, not vision. The old structure remains in Wordsworth, but it has undergone a true sea-change.

Wordsworth likewise resembles Boccaccio in his abhorrence for cities, his insistence that uninterrupted meditation must precede composition, and his locating the meditative act in the simplicity of the countryside. Boccaccio, for example, venerates Nature with a Wordsworthian fervor. Consider the following passage:

> There the beeches stretch themselves, with other trees, toward heaven; there they spread a thick shade with their fresh green foliage; there the earth is covered with grass and dotted with flowers of a thousand colors; there, too, are clear fountains and argent brooks that fall with a gentle murmur

[2] Ibid., p. 744a.

from the mountain's breast. There are gay song-birds, and the boughs stirred to a soft sound by the wind, and playful little animals; and there the flocks and herds, the shepherd's cottage or the little hut untroubled with domestic cares; and all is filled with peace and quiet. Then, as these pleasures possess both eye and ear, they soothe the soul; then they collect the scattered energies of the mind, and renew the power of the poet's genius, if it be weary, prompting it, as it were, to long for contemplation of high themes, and yearn for expression—

[GDC 14. 11]

Nature was certainly no discovery of the Romantic poets. The allegorist needed her healing powers for his own inspiration.

In his conception of the poet's subject matter, Wordsworth again suggests parallels with the allegorists. In the *Preface* he argues that the object of poetry is Truth, which he defines as an "image of man and nature."[3] The allegorical critic would have said this slightly differently. Poetry ultimately contains psychological and cosmological truth. Characteristically, Wordsworth slants this definition toward the psychological. Poetry unites men to the world, for it makes the world warm or alive through the projecting power of the mind.[4] Wordsworth is not so certain that man and Nature invariably go together. Descartes had already killed the external world and isolated man from it, so Wordsworth reunites the two through poetry. The allegorist had no such doubts. Man by his very nature reflects the cosmos and poetry expresses this relationship. Poetry need not create it.

Wordsworth's version of the old structure, although less self-assured, gave him certain advantages never allowed to a Renaissance allegorist. For example, he could accept an oratorical conception of language and avoid the old problem of obscurity altogether. His poet has no superhuman truth to express, nothing far beyond the normal thought-modes of his audience. He describes the appearances of things, the pictures painted on the veil,

[3] Ibid., p. 737b.
[4] M. H. Abrams, *The Mirror and the Lamp* (New York, 1958), p. 64.

not the Truth shining through it.[5] His purpose is to voice his passion, and, insofar as he relies on certain ideas, he works *within* the commonplaces of his audience. There is no reason then why he cannot communicate his experiences directly to others, and plain language best accomplishes this purpose. Wordsworth can, therefore, adopt the principle of clarity with all its implications, something Spenser never could have done. In fact, Wordsworth strove as hard as Ben Jonson had done to reform and simplify the language of poetry. The Temple once more had to be cleansed.

Wordsworth devoted a great portion of his famous *Preface* plus an Appendix to the question of poetic diction, and there he repeated many tenets familiar to an oratorical critic of the Renaissance. He argued strongly for a clear and plain language in poetry and equaled a Daniel or Jonson in his suspicion of poetic diction. The pleasure of it, he said, rests primarily "in impressing a notion of the peculiarity and exaltation of the Poet's character, and in flattering the Reader's self-love by bringing him nearer to a sympathy with that character."[6]

Again, as one would expect, Wordsworth does not distinguish the language of poetry from that of prose except to say that it represents a careful selection from normal idiom and is arranged metrically. He discusses meter extensively, of course, and provides a justification for it, replacing Puttenham's cosmic explanation with a psychological one. In typical fashion he goes on to say that this plain language is designed for an unspecialized audience, and he explicitly excludes the professions, just as Puttenham had: "The Poet writes under one restriction only, namely, the necessity of giving immediate pleasure to a human Being possessed of that information which may be expected from him, not as a lawyer, a physician, a mariner, an astronomer, or a natural philosopher, but as a Man."[7] Both Wordsworth and Puttenham think in

[5] Wordsworth, p. 743a.

[6] Ibid., p. 742a.

[7] Ibid., p. 737b.

terms of an orator's audience and they both emphasize pleasure as the pragmatic end or condition of poetry. In one place Wordsworth even brings in the Horatian ends of pleasure and profit, and he allows the audience judgment over the poet, as must any orator, though he limits its exercise to lifelong students of poetry. Jonson had gone one step further and allowed judgment only to other poets. In matters of language Wordsworth upholds the oratorical and neoclassical tradition.

But he upholds it with a difference of emphasis. Wordsworth is less concerned with the poet's audience than he is with the poet himself, and he advocates clear language primarily because it expresses the poet's feelings more directly. For the same reasons he violates classical precedent and uses rustic language as the model for his style rather than the language of London and the Court. Rustics express their emotions without verbal pretensions, and Wordsworth believes that their emotions, being simpler, can be more accurately described and communicated.[8] Herbert had thought, rather, that country people lacked sensibility, an idea which Coleridge applied to Wordsworth, when he argued that rural life causes grossness instead of excellence of feeling.[9] Wordsworth is wrong here, but Coleridge's criticism should not be allowed to hide the reorientation of Wordsworth's classicism. The poet speaks less to the capacity of his hearers than to his interior emotional state. And it is here that Wordsworth's conception of language reflects his allegorical model. Neoclassic he may be in specific questions, but the governing control in his theory is not oratorical but allegorical. The poet's feelings overflow and fill his audience with the same experiences. Wordsworth's disagreement with Spenser would be over what language best suited this purpose, not over the purpose itself.

In one sense Sir Philip Sidney provides the best Renaissance parallel to Wordsworth. They both mediated between oratorical

8 Ibid., p. 735a.
9 Abrams, p. 120.

and prophetic rhetoric, and they could do so because they both thought of the poet psychologically, as a unique genius. Their explanations differed widely: the one talked of wit, the other of imagination and passion. In either case, however, clarity of language became a virtue, while many allegorical notions of poetry could still be retained; and perhaps it was for that reason that they were so influential. Modern critics can use Sidney to interpret both Spenser and Jonson; and Harington, though an allegorist, regarded Sidney's *Defence* with high approval. Similarly, Wordsworth's influence can be found everywhere, both among his contemporaries and ever since. The mean always draws more followers than the extremes.

II
Shelley

In his *Defence of Poetry* Shelley presupposes the same structure of poetic experience which we have found in Wordsworth and the Renaissance allegorists. He goes further than Wordsworth, however, and revives practically the whole of allegorical theory, including its linguistic basis. Our discussion of Shelley, therefore, will read rather like a summary of this book—its logical conclusion.

I will begin with language. Shelley says of poets that "their language is vitally metaphorical; that is, it marks the before unapprehended relations of things and perpetuates their apprehension."[10] In the Renaissance poetry was identified with allegory, itself a continued metaphor. And like the allegorist Shelley gives for meter the same explanation which he used for metaphor. Both meter and metaphor signify a perception of order in relations. The allegorist would have talked about memory and judg-

---

[10] *The Selected Poetry and Prose of Percy Bysshe Shelley*, ed. Carlos Baker (New York, 1951), p. 496. Most of this discussion is based on his *Defence*.

ment, but he would have agreed with Shelley in considering both figured language and rhythmic pattern as varieties of the same thing. In regard to the poet himself Shelley revives in full the theory of divine inspiration. Poetry has divine origins, for it brings light and power from eternal regions where the calculating faculty never dares soar.[11] Within the poet inspiration acts unconsciously, for the mind in creation is fired by an invisible influence. The Muse *dictated* to Milton his "unpremeditated song." While under the Muse's control, the poet thinks outside of time and experiences an ecstasy in which his sense of self diminishes to nothing. Like Spenser, Shelley's *vates* approaches his art with due humility, for he is a vehicle of power, not its cause. His own poems represent feeble echoes of the original vision. The *poema* exists to stimulate vision, not as an end in itself. Borrowing the old mystery language once more, Shelley concludes that "Poets are the hierophants of an unapprehended inspiration."[12]

In the *Defence* Shelley does not speak directly of the necessity for obscurantist rhetoric, but he does envisage the poet as singing alone, unattentive to any audience. He develops the obscurantist side of this notion in his allegory about poetry, *The Witch of Atlas*, itself composed under inspiration within three days. The Witch, who is poetic truth and beauty, finds that she must veil her face:

> For she was beautiful—her beauty made
> The bright world dim, and everything beside
> Seemed like the fleeting image of a shade:
> No thought of living spirit could abide,
> Which to her looks had ever been betrayed,
> On any object in the world so wide,
> On any hope within the circling skies,
> But on her form, and in her inmost eyes.

[11] Ibid., p. 517.
[12] Ibid., p. 522.

Which when the lady knew, she took her spindle
  And twined three threads of fleecy mist, and three
Long lines of light, such as the dawn may kindle
  The clouds and waves and mountains with; and she
As many star-beams, ere their lamps could dwindle
  In the belated moon, wound skilfully;
And with these threads a subtle veil she wove—
A shadow for the splendour of her love.

[12-13]

Boccaccio had used the same explanation, replacing beauty with truth, which, of course, are the same in a Platonizing system. In *Prometheus Unbound* Shelley presents another view of the same situation. Asia and Panthea ride to a cloudy mountain top. Panthea observes that, though the sun has not yet risen, the cloud radiates light. The Spirit of the Hour explains that Asia once more is shining in her full glory, as she had done when the sea gave her birth, and Panthea admits that she cannot look upon her sister. She feels rather than sees the heart of light. Or in Boccaccio's terms, the truth of allegory can sometimes be so profound that it will blind the critic, even when clearly presented and unveiled. The critic's human limitations create his own veil. He cannot gaze directly upon the sun (*GDG* 14. 12). Immediately afterward, a chorus of Spirits from *outside* the cloud hymn Asia's beauty shining *through* the cloud. This is the normal situation in allegory, where the artist deliberately veils truth and his audience perceives it indirectly. As Boccaccio explains it, on a cloudy day one can perceive the radiance of the sun but not its exact position. The veil remains, whether one is within or without the cloud. This fact provides Shelley with his famous definition of poetry in the *Defence*, and it would have pleased a Renaissance allegorist. All high poetry is infinite, for no one will ever strip away the veils from the beauty of meaning. He then uses the age-old metaphor of the nut, transposing the image into the Romantic growing plant, but with the same signification. The allegorist peels off the outer bark of the nut, looking for the concealed truth. Shelley thinks of a great poem as an acorn becoming an oak tree, meaning something different to every succeeding age. Poetry escapes the limits of time and its symbols are ever relevant, just as the poet thinks within a timeless world.

Shelley differs from his Renaissance predecessors in his definition of this truth or beauty. He argues that the object of poetry is the eternal forms of human nature as they exist in the Mind of the Creator, which itself images all other minds. An allegorist would agree with this statement but would add that a poem images the cosmos as well, which also shadows the divine *mens*. Shelley can talk of the earth in these terms—witness the famous analogy of the glass dome in Adonais—but he does not put the two ideas together, unless he does so in a lyric from *Prometheus*, where he says of the poet:

> He will watch from dawn to gloom
> The lake-reflected sun illume
> The yellow bees in the ivy-bloom,
> Nor heed nor see, what things they be;
> But from these create he can
> Forms more real than living man,
> Nurslings of immortality!
>
> [1. 743-49]

In any case, the emphasis again is away from the cosmological and toward the psychological, as in Wordsworth. The Renaissance critic would have agreed enthusiastically, however, with Shelley's distinction between mere fiction and poetry. The one catalogs facts, the other reveals the eternal forms behind the facts.[13] Boccaccio said much the same thing. A story without depth or levels of meaning is an old wives' tale, not a poem.

Unlike his predecessors, Shelley did not conclude that divine truth necessitated a dual audience for the poet. He never thought about the problem, and in this respect the Romantics talked more radically than the old allegorists. The poet sings alone and devotes himself completely to his inward truth. Any attention to

13 Ibid., p. 499.

an audience would destroy his poetry and turn it into mere rhetoric. The poet cannot serve two masters, his own truth and the requirements of his audience. The technological revolution of the preceding centuries might explain this change. In 1800 poetry was read and had ceased to be regarded as a living oral art. The Renaissance allegorist could not ignore his audience, for it was part of his very conception of poetry. Not so the Romantics.

Otherwise, Shelley repeats the old commonplaces about the poet's audience. Poetry communicates wisdom through delight;[14] it creates the moral values of society. Shelley says that the Greeks imitated Homer's mythic figures, and Spenser had tried to stimulate the same kind of imitation among his contemporaries. The poet is a euhemeristic educator, the fountain of society and religion. His moral power, though, is explained differently. The Renaissance critic thought of it linguistically: morality inevitably followed from tropological discourse. Shelley, as one would expect, thinks of the matter psychologically. The imagination is the perception of value in the quantities which Reason knows. The result is the same in either case. Society mirrors poetry. It follows from this euhemerism that society and poetry are mutually interdependent. A decline in one coincides with a decline in the other. Neither Spenser nor Shelley can conceive of poetry as distinct from the moral condition of their contemporaries. The poet both creates morality and is its victim.

A significant difference, however, does separate Shelley from the old allegorists, but it is not an easy thing to point out. One way of saying it might be that the Romantics substituted imagination for memory. Shelley constantly stresses the *creative* power of the poetic imagination. The poet makes a new morality: he widens the imagination of man and allows him to perceive new relationships. Through this extension of the imagination love becomes possible, and love is the secret of morals.[15] Spenser, on the contrary, did not create values but recalled old ones to his

14 Ibid., p. 500.
15 Ibid., pp. 501-2.

audience, values now almost forgotten. Blake would call Spenser's poetry a fable or allegory made by the daughters of Memory, a form which he contemptuously contrasts with Vision or Imagination, surrounded by the daughters of Inspiration.[16] But this clear-cut distinction breaks down on closer investigation. Too many Romantics depended upon memory. Byron wrote from personal memories, and Wordsworth made memory an essential part of poetic creation. Pragmatically, little separates the poet who recalls forgotten values and the visionary who creates new ones for a society. In both cases these values appear new to that society. The contrast between memory and imagination does not explain the difference between the two periods, but it illuminates a shift in emphasis. The Romantic tends to look forward into the future, while the Renaissance poet dreams of the past. It is the difference between Spenser's nostalgic tale of medieval knights and ladies and Shelley's eschatological myth, *Prometheus Unbound*.

A critic might describe the difference more fundamentally by contrasting the Renaissance and Romantic conceptions of truth. Shelley's poet perceives not Platonic Ideas shining through the veil of the material cosmos but relations—between existence and perception, between perception and expression.[17] His truth is primarily psychological, of the associational type developed in the eighteenth century. A Renaissance critic would consider this definition too subjective. It leaves no room for objective truth, and the cosmos dwindles into an aspect of the psyche. We have already seen how Wordsworth slanted his theory in a psychological direction, and Shelley does it too. He parallels all his Platonic *dicta* with psychological reinterpretations. From a Renaissance standpoint this persistent psychologizing shuts up the poet within himself and cuts him off from the world and ultimately from truth. Wordsworth limits his poet to a description of appearances, to the pictures on the veil; that is, his poet does not

16 Blake, p. 386.
17 Shelley, p. 496.

write allegory at all. Shelley in an early sonnet, "Lift not the painted veil," seems to advocate the same position. The man who looked behind the veil came away disappointed. No truth was to be found there.

But this distinction breaks down too because it ignores the Romantics' historical situation. Copernicus and Descartes had killed the old cosmos. What remained was a dead machine, separated from the living minds of men. Wordsworth's poet healed the breach. Through the projecting power of his imagination, the poet revivified Nature and united it to man. The external world became a veil through which shone the poet's passion and sensibility. And, as in the Renaissance, the poet's inward state absolutely depended upon this cosmic veil for its value. Boccaccio had said that the poets veil truth so that they may valorize it in the minds of others (*GDG* 14. 12). Clement describes the process more precisely. Sunlight reveals the defects in an object, but fruit in water or figures behind veils have added reflections. They look grander and more imposing (*Strom.* 5. 9). Similarly, the Romantic critics recognized the value of the poet's veil. Shelley's bold "Spirit" in the sonnet made a crucial mistake, for he looked behind the veil rather than through it. Such a revelation was reserved instead for those like Asia and Panthea, who descended through the volcanic vapour, "Through the cloudy strife/Of Death and of Life" (2. 3. 57-58), to perceive the imageless truth beyond the veil, the formless darkness of Demogorgon. Death alone removes the veil. Apuleius' votary experienced a simulated death before he saw the eternal powers, and, in *Adonais*, Shelley explicitly places the eternal forms beyond the limits of human life. And even then he is looking through a veil:

> The breath whose might I have invoked in song
> Descends on me; my spirit's bark is driven,
> Far from the shore, far from the trembling throng
> Whose sails were never to the tempest given;
> The massy earth and sphered skies are riven!
> I am borne darkly, fearfully, afar;

> Whilst, burning *through the inmost veil* of Heaven,
> The soul of Adonais, like a star,
> Beacons from the abode where the Eternal are.
>
> [487-95; italics mine]

One must say that allegory did in fact revive among some of the Romantics, but at the same time one must add that the understanding of allegory had altered, sometimes radically. The allegorists' structuring of the poetic process reappeared, but not always the content. And yet this structure had tremendous influence on all the Romantics. It jostled with neoclassicism in Wordsworth's *Preface* and survived—all the way up to the twentieth century. Eliot's objective correlative is just another version of the same structure. Like institutions, allegory never really dies. It may adopt a new terminology and defend itself in the current educated idiom, but its form remains—which is an appropriate fate for a Platonizing system.

Index